THE ADVENTIST
HEALTHSTYLE

THE ADVENTIST HEALTHSTYLE

David C. Nieman, D.H.Sc., M.P.H., F.A.C.S.M.

REVIEW AND HERALD® PUBLISHING ASSOCIATION
HAGERSTOWN, MD 21740

The author assumes full responsibility for the accuracy of all facts and quotations as cited in this book.

Texts credited to NEB are from *The New English Bible*. © The Delegates of the Oxford University Press and the Syndics of the Cambridge University Press 1962, 1970. Reprinted by permission.

Texts credited to NIV are from the *Holy Bible, New International Version*. Copyright © 1973, 1978, 1984, International Bible Society. Used by permission of Zondervan Bible Publishers.

Verses marked TLB are taken from *The Living Bible,* copyright © 1971 by Tyndale House Publishers, Wheaton, Ill. Used by permission.

This book was
Edited by Barbara Jackson-Hall
Designed by Bill Kirstein
Cover photos by Tom Radcliffe; inset by David Brownell
Typeset: 11/12 Times Roman

PRINTED IN U.S.A.

97 96 95 94 93 92   10 9 8 7 6 5 4 3 2 1

Library of Congress Cataloging in Publication Data
Nieman, David C., 1950-
   The Adventist healthstyle / David C. Nieman.
     p. cm.

   1. Health—Religious aspects—Seventh-day Adventists. 2. Seventh-day Adventists—Doctrines. 3. Adventists—Doctrines. I. Title.
BX6154.N593 1992
261.8'321—dc20   92-11513
                                  CIP

ISBN 0-8280-0657-1

Dedication

To my mother, Anna Nieman, who has taught me through her example the true meaning of God's love.

Contents

Introduction

Near the end of the apostle John's life, he wrote a short personal letter to Gaius, a faithful Christian who is highly commended for his hospitality to itinerant preachers and teachers. In this letter, which we now know as 3 John, two other characters are mentioned by John: Diotrephes, a church leader who was stirring up some trouble by his contentious actions; and Demetrius, probably a traveling teacher. The apostle's authority was being undermined by the Diotrephes faction, and John wrote a simple and direct letter to Gaius to ensure the delivery of his message to the loyal church members.

A spirit of tender personal attention is evident in John's letter, and perhaps because of the stress and anxiety that all may have been feeling, he starts by writing, "Dear friend, I pray that you may enjoy good health and that all may go well with you, even as your soul is getting along well" (3 John 2, NIV).

Two major thoughts are expressed here. John's heartfelt prayer is that Gaius may have general prosperity, both spiritually and materially. John also appears concerned about Gaius' health and wishes that it, too, may be as good as his strong spiritual life.

This book, *The Adventist Healthstyle*, is patterned after this prayer and concern of John's. The book is divided into 13 chapters, with each written to broaden the content found in the 13 lessons of the *Adult Sabbath School Quarterly* entitled "Look Up and Live."

A special attempt has been made to bring you up-to-date on the latest scientific findings on important health issues. The style of the book is informative, yet philosophical and anecdotal. It is the sincere desire of the author and publishers that *The Adventist Healthstyle* will aid you in your plans for good health as you walk the path of life.

CHAPTER 1

The Meaning
of Health

*"The 'positiveness' of health does not lie
in the state, but in the struggle—the effort
to reach a goal which in its perfection
is unattainable."*—Lancet 2 (1958): 638.

D r. Bernie Siegel describes in his book *Love, Medicine,
and Miracles* (New York: Harper and Row Publishers,
1986) an experience he had with Jonathan, a physician
who had just been diagnosed as having lung cancer. He had been
admitted into the hospital in relatively good physical and mental
condition. When he learned of his diagnosis, however, he
became terribly depressed and withdrawn. Although Dr. Siegel
attempted to elevate his spirit and attitude, Jonathan remained
disconsolate and died two weeks later. Jonathan's wife thanked
Dr. Siegel for his efforts, but explained that her husband hadn't
wanted to fight for recovery. Just prior to his demise, he had
remarked to her that his life and work had lost all meaning.

The ancient Greek physician Hippocrates once wrote that he
would rather know what sort of person has a disease than what
sort of disease a person has. Sir William Osler, a famous
Canadian physician during the late 1800s, argued that the
outcome of tuberculosis had more to do with what went on in the
patient's mind than what went on in his lungs.

Although it has long been felt by many health professionals
that mental, social, and spiritual factors have much to do with an
individual's health and well-being, modern medicine seldom

emphasizes these components in actual practice. As Dr. Siegel has written: "Practitioners still act as though disease catches people, rather than understanding that people catch disease by becoming susceptible to the seeds of illness to which we are all constantly exposed."

In this chapter we will review the true meaning of health from both a biblical and a scientific viewpoint. Just what is health? What are its domains?

Health in the Bible

When Jesus invited Matthew the tax collector to "follow Me," Matthew responded joyfully by organizing a great banquet for many of his colleagues and friends, including Jesus. When the all-too-predictable Pharisees complained to His disciples, Jesus responded by saying, "It is not the healthy [*hugiaino*] who need a doctor, but the sick. I have not come to call the righteous, but sinners to repentance" (Luke 5:31, NIV).

The Greek word *hugiaino* comes from *hugiés*, a Greek term for health, soundness, and wholeness. Paul repeatedly uses the same word, applying it to "sound doctrine" (1 Timothy 1:10), "sound" words (2 Timothy 1:13), and being "sound" in the faith (Titus 1:13). Perhaps the most popular use of the term in the Bible is found in the verse where John writes, "Beloved, I wish above all things that thou mayest prosper and be in health, even as thy soul prospereth" (3 John 2, KJV). In *The New English Bible* this verse reads: "My dear Gaius, I pray that you may enjoy good health, and that all may go well with you, as I know it goes well with your soul."

Throughout Scripture health is intimately tied to both mental and spiritual well-being. This is most evident in the Psalms. For example, in Psalm 6, often interpreted as David's anguish over his son Absalom, we read the words, "O Lord, heal me, for my bones are in agony. My soul is in anguish" (verses 2, 3, NIV). The psalm of the cross, Psalm 22, graphically portrays this theme, as does Psalm 31:

"Be merciful to me, O Lord, for I am in distress; my eyes

grow weak with sorrow, my soul and my body with grief. My life is consumed by anguish and my years by groaning; my strength fails because of my affliction, and my bones grow weak'' (Psalm 31:9,10, NIV).

In Proverbs, Solomon repeatedly delineates the health advantages that come through knowing and loving God.

"My son, do not forget my teaching, but keep my commands in your heart, for they will prolong your life many years and bring you prosperity.'' "Do not be wise in your own eyes; fear the Lord and shun evil. This will bring health to your body and nourishment to your bones'' (Proverbs 3:1, 2, 7, 8, NIV).

"My son, pay attention to what I say; listen closely to my words. Do not let them out of your sight, keep them within your heart; for they are life to those who find them and health to a man's whole body'' (Proverbs 4:20-22, NIV).

"The fear of the Lord is a fountain of life. . . . A heart at peace gives life to the body, but envy rots the bones'' (Proverbs 14:27-30, NIV).

In *The Ministry of Healing*, the health classic by Ellen G. White, a constant theme is the deep-seated relationship between physical, mental, and spiritual health.

"From Him flowed a stream of healing power, and in body and mind and soul men were made whole'' (p. 17).

"Whatever injures the health not only lessens physical vigor, but tends to weaken the mental and moral powers'' (p. 128).

"The relation that exists between the mind and the body is very intimate. When one is affected, the other sympathizes. . . . Courage, hope, faith, sympathy, love, promote health and prolong life'' (p. 241).

The Meaning of Health in the World Today

The most notable, and undoubtedly still the most influential, definition of health is that of the World Health Organization. The definition appeared in the preamble of its constitution during the late 1940s:

"Health is a state of complete physical, mental, and social well-being, and not merely the absence of disease and infirmity."

This definition stemmed from a conviction of WHO organizers that the security of future world peace would lie in the improvement of physical, mental, and social health. The definition suggests that health goes beyond the mere avoidance of disease and extends to how one feels and functions physically, mentally, and socially. Absent from the definition is any mention of a spiritual component. Perhaps the WHO organizers felt that some nations would object to any mention of or emphasis on spiritual health.

Physical health has usually been defined as the absence of disease and disability, while having sufficient energy and vitality to accomplish daily tasks and active recreational pursuits without undue fatigue. Social health refers to the ability to interact effectively with other people and the social environment, engaging in satisfying personal relationships. There is good evidence that people who have many social ties to others experience less disease and greater feelings of well-being.

Mental or psychological health refers to both the absence of mental disorders and the ability of the individual to negotiate the daily challenges and social interactions of life without experiencing mental, emotional, or behavioral functional problems. Later in this book, we will review the mounting evidence that psychological well-being has much to do with one's physical health (see chapters 10 and 11).

Despite this evidence, many physicians still are not convinced that the brain can exert measurable effects on the body. For example, in April of 1990, Dr. Redford Williams, writing for the *Journal of the American Medical Association,* described that "there is still skepticism that mental states—and, hence, the brain—play an important role in physical illness, with some in positions of authority consigning such a notion to the realm of 'folklore.' " Dr. Williams goes on to explain that much of the brain-body research is inconsistent, and that many researchers are reluctant to get into this line of investigation.

What About Spiritual Health?

There is even more resistance when the relationship between spiritual matters and physical health is considered. In fact, there are relatively few published research articles in this area.

There are several reasons for this. First and foremost is that spiritual factors are very difficult to gauge. Science likes to measure relevant factors in an objective way, and this is not easy to do when it comes to spiritual concerns. No one has yet determined just which spiritual factors should be considered, or how they can be defined and precisely measured.

Second, spiritual issues tend to be seen as very personal. Some health researchers are quite reluctant to measure spiritual factors in their subjects because they are afraid of "turning them off," or creating unnecessary obstacles.

Another reason for the lack of scientific data in the area of spiritual health is that modern-day Western culture is dominated largely by an interest in materialism rather than spirituality. Many researchers just don't care about spiritual factors or are unconvinced that they're important.

With these reasons in mind, it should come as no surprise that scientific literature contains scant references to spiritual matters.

To give you an example of some of the problems involved in measuring spiritual health, consider a recent study by a group of researchers in Jerusalem. Dr. Yechiel Friedlander of the Hadassah University Hospital has published several studies looking at the relationship between religious observance and coronary heart disease in Jewish residents of Jerusalem.

He has reported that Jewish subjects who were more secular experienced greater rates of heart disease and had more of the typical risk factors than did the more orthodox subjects. In other words, the greater the degree of religious observance in the

Jewish subjects, the less they suffered from heart disease. Other studies have also found that "religiosity" is protective against coronary heart disease.

As you might suspect, however, some Christians do not regard religious observance as the best indicator of spiritual health. They see one's relationship with God and aptitude to serve others in love as the real determinants. The Pharisees of Christ's day provide the best example of this. People who are "religious" may be more willing to live in a healthy manner, and so any health advantage may be related to their superior health habits, not spiritual health.

In an ideal study, the first step would be to locate a large group of atheists and randomly divide them into two groups. Those in the control group would continue their atheistic ways. Those in the experimental group would begin a walk with God. After a long period of time (at least 20 years), the two groups would be compared for a wide variety of health and death measures to see if the "spiritual" group experienced any advantage.

You can imagine the terrible time researchers would have in conducting this study (for instance, deciding just how the experimental group should live and how it would be measured). And how many atheists do you think would volunteer for the study? Obviously this study will never be done.

A few published studies do provide some interesting findings. One of the better studies to date was conducted by Dr. Melvin Pollner from the University of California at Los Angeles. In his paper entitled "Divine Relations, Social Relations, and Well-being," Dr. Pollner reports his findings from the 1983 and 1984 General Social Survey. In the study, more than 3,000 Americans were questioned on various aspects of social and religious behavior, beliefs, and images of God (*Journal of Health and Social Behavior* 30 [1989]: 92-104).

Dr. Pollner points out that growing evidence indicates persons who have many social relations (supportive family and friends), tend to experience higher levels of both mental and physical well-being than persons who have few. He also reasons that alongside an individual's "real" social network exists a network of "imagined others." These include unmet, unmeetable, or imaginary people drawn from the popular media, history, and religion (e.g., movie stars, past presidents, Old Testament figures, etc.).

Recent Gallup surveys show that 87 percent of adult Americans pray to God; 69 percent feel that God has guided them in making decisions; and 36 percent feel that God has spoken directly to them through some means.

Eighty percent of American adults feel at least "somewhat close" to God most of the time; 47 percent report that they have experienced a spiritual force that seemed to lift them out of themselves.

Based on these surveys, Dr. Pollner reasons that many Americans participate in "divine relations" as well as social relations and that divine relationships may be just as meaningful to their psychological well-being as the real social ones that people engage in on a daily basis.

In the General Social Survey, people were asked such questions as: "How close do you feel to God most of the time?" "About how often do you pray?" "How often have you felt as though you were very close to a powerful, spiritual force that seemed to lift you out of yourself?" In addition to these and other questions on church attendance, education, and income, study participants filled in the General Well-being psychological questionnaire.

After a thorough statistical analysis, Dr. Pollner concluded that "participation in a divine relation is the strongest correlate . . . of well-being, surpassing in strength such usually potent predictors as race, sex, income, age, marital status, and church attendance. . . . Whatever the mediating processes prove to be, they are as potent as virtually any that affect well-being." In other words, one's relationship with God is strongly associated with psychological well-being.

It is hoped that this interesting study will spur many other researchers to devote time and effort toward exploring this issue further. Many questions remain to be answered.

Defining Spiritual Health

Important questions for scientists who wish to conduct research along the lines of what Dr. Pollner did are: 1. What is spiritual health? 2. How do you measure it? 3. Can a clear improvement in overall health (not just psychological well-being) be measured in those who have spiritual health versus those who don't? In other words, can you have good health without possessing spiritual health? 4. Is there a special advantage in being a Christian versus a Jew or a Muslim?

Recently, in a bold and fresh departure from most health-medical journals, the *American Journal of Health Promotion* defined optimal health as "a balance of physical, emotional, social, spiritual, and intellectual health" (3, No. 3 [1989]: 5). Several articles on spiritual health have been published by this journal, and a definition has been proposed:

"Optimal spiritual health is defined as the ability to develop one's spiritual nature to its fullest potential. This includes our ability: to discover, articulate, and act on our own basic purpose in life; to learn how to give and receive love, joy, and peace; to pursue a fulfilling life; and to contribute to the improvement of the spiritual health of others" (1, No. 2 [1987]: 12-17).

This journal takes the stance that man does have a spiritual dimension, and that health professionals should address this domain in their day-to-day contacts with patients and clients, while avoiding "religious proselytizing, singular theism, or dogmatism. . . . We may have limited our theories of human possibility through the exclusion of spirituality" (5, No. 4 [1991]: 273-281).

Various spiritual health skills are listed by the journal, including self-awareness, self-inquiry, search for knowledge, behavior change, cognitive restructuring, relational skills, life goal planning, and lifestyle management. Health professionals are urged by the journal to administer spiritual assessment questionnaires to patients and small groups, and then discuss responses. Various "spiritual health interventions" can then follow, including development of "personal scenarios" such as having participants write their own obituaries, or a brief outline of their own biography, or actual/expected major life goals at each stage of life. Questions such as "What characterizes a 'successful life'?" or "How much fulfillment should you have in your life?" or "What things give meaning to life?" or "What determines the quality of our lives?" can be asked in small group settings to invoke discussion.

What Does Belief in Christ Add?

As you might suspect by now, this approach to improving the spiritual health of individuals is generic, without any emphasis on developing a relationship with Christ. Obviously this is unacceptable to most Christians, but in the very least, such an approach could be used as a starting point.

It will be interesting to see where scientific research will lead us in the future. It is possible that researchers will conclude that belief in any deity or religion may result in close to the same health benefits. In other words, it is not so much what you believe in as it is the process of belief. How would you handle such a finding?

While we are on this earth as pilgrims (Hebrews 11:13), there are many health habits that we can adopt to make our sojourn a bit easier, more productive, and less painful. From the diet we choose to the God we trust, all are important. However, God may have decided that the individual walking in the opposite direction can also enjoy relatively good health despite lack of complete trust in Him. The tragic difference, however, is that one enters into eternal life, while the other doesn't. There is no greater health benefit than this—eternal life—and everything else pales in comparison.

Christ has made it very plain that knowing Him is the only way for mankind to experience complete peace and joy, and eternal life (John 3:16, 11:25, 26; 14:6). Abraham Lincoln once wrote that "we were designed by God to trust in Him." In other words, only as we meet our God-given design by depending on and trusting in Him will we experience complete health and fulfillment.

A life without a relationship with God will result in less-than-desirable health and satisfaction because function must follow design. For example, the human body is designed for motion, and only if we exercise can we feel good, be healthy, and avoid early death from various diseases (see chapter 5). The same is true regarding our inherent design and need to trust in God.

Health has been called a mirage. You can reach for it, but never fully grasp it. Health is not so much a possession as a procession; not so much something to have as it is a way to be. A person can never say "I am healthy." Instead, he or she is always within the process, seeking to attain a goal that is in itself unattainable.

The parallel to the spiritual life is striking. We can never say that we "have arrived" spiritually until Christ takes us home to live with Him for eternity. Christ is our Creator and Redeemer, and how foolish it is for anyone to tread the path of life without Him.

CHAPTER 2

Disease Prevention

---

*"To ward off disease or recover health, men
as a rule find it easier to depend on the
healers than to attempt the more difficult
task of living wisely."—Rene Dubos.*

Folk wisdom holds that an ounce of prevention is worth a pound of cure. But most people would rather quote this statement or agree with it in theory than put it into practice.

British prime minister Winston Churchill said it well on a visit to his personal physician because of headaches, wheezing, aches, pains, and shortness of breath. "You've got to stop smoking a dozen cigars a day and staying up half the night drinking a bottle of cognac," his doctor admonished. "If I wanted to do that," Churchill shot back, "I wouldn't need you."

John Knowles, the late president of the Rockefeller Foundation, wrote in 1977, "Over 99 percent of us are born healthy and are made sick as a result of personal misbehaviors and environmental conditions."

Dr. Ken Cooper of the Aerobic Institute in Dallas, Texas, is fond of saying that "we don't die of a disease anymore, we die because of the way we live."

Dr. Walter Bortz in his book *We Live Too Short and Die Too Long* (New York: Bantam Books, 1991) tells the story of a patient of his, a 63-year-old box manufacturer from Red Bluff, California, whom he had seen a year earlier for a complete physical examination. "My notations revealed that he had come into my office preceded considerably by his belly. He was red-faced, angry, and smoking heavily. Furthermore, he had high blood pressure and a very elevated cholesterol level. His face twitched. His chest heaved. A time bomb waiting to go off." Now the patient was returning for another appointment, and Dr. Bortz was expecting the worst. Instead, a slim, energetic man walked into his office. He had lost 60 pounds, stopped smoking, and was jogging five miles a day. Writes Dr. Bortz, "His blood pressure was normal. His cholesterol was low. . . . I had nothing to do with it. He had, in a secret, quiet moment, looked into the mirror and not liked what he saw. His transformation cost nothing, involved neither drugs, hospitals, nor technologies. He simply decided to link up with a better future. . . . Of course, I was ecstatic. Such dramatic representations occur seldom, but often enough to sustain my conviction that prevention is where the action is—or should be" (pp. 68, 69).

Old Testament Principles

According to the 1850 census of the leading causes of death, 60 percent of all deaths in the United States were caused by infectious diseases, including, in order of importance, tuberculosis, dysentery and diarrhea, cholera, malaria, typhoid fever, pneumonia, diphtheria, scarlet fever, meningitis, whooping cough, measles, erysipelas, and smallpox.

The great proportion of these deaths were the result of polluted water supplies, inadequate sewage disposal, polluted milk and food, overcrowding, little protection from flies and other insects that spread disease, poor nutrition, long hours of overwork, and gross ignorance and carelessness. Most of these infectious diseases have largely been controlled in Western countries as a result of cleaner water, milk, and food supplies, upgrades in the standard of living and housing, immunization, improvement in garbage and sewage disposal, and health education. However, other infectious diseases have sprung up in their place, notably sexually transmitted diseases and AIDS, both of which are associated with having more than one sexual partner (more will be said on these diseases later in this chapter).

Although modern medicine has successfully learned how to prevent the most devastating of the infectious diseases, similar success has not been experienced for today's major causes of death, particularly coronary heart disease, cancer, and stroke, which together account for some 70 percent of all deaths in the United States. These diseases have been called "lifestyle diseases," or chronic diseases, because they are very much related to the way we eat, our exercise habits, body weight, use of tobacco and alcohol, and stress levels.

Several health principles from the Old Testament pertaining to sanitation, diet, and sexual behavior apply to both infectious and lifestyle disease prevention. Mankind's original diet was to come totally from the plant kingdom (Genesis 1:29, 30; 3:18).

Men and women strayed from this ideal, however, and God laid down several safeguards for the Hebrew people when they desired to include meat in their diets. No blood or fat from the animal was to be consumed (Leviticus 3:17; 7:22-27; 17:10-14; 1 Samuel 2:16) which decreased the level of saturated fat and cholesterol intake, greatly decreasing their risk of heart disease and cancer. People who completely avoided intake of alcohol were to be held in high esteem (Numbers 6:3, 4; Judges 13:4).

Many rules for sanitation were given, including the burial of human excreta (Deuteronomy 23:13-15), procedures to prevent foodstuffs from contamination or spoilage (Exodus 16:19; Leviticus 11:31-40; 19:5-8), proper disposal of animal parts not eaten (Leviticus 4:11, 12), personal bathing and washing of garments (Genesis 35:2; Exodus 19:10; Leviticus 15, 17:15, 16; Jeremiah 2:22; Ecclesiastes 9:8), quarantine for those with major infectious skin diseases (Leviticus 13, 14; Numbers 5:2-4), and sterilization of war booty obtained from other nations (Numbers 31:21-24). Each of these rules safeguarded the spread of infectious diseases among the Israelite people.

God made it plain that husband and wife were not to commit adultery and were to have sexual relations only with their spouse

(Genesis 2:24; Exodus 20:14; Leviticus 18:1-22; 20:10-21). Sexual relations with animals were also prohibited (Exodus 22:19; Leviticus 18:23; 20:15, 16). These rules would prevent the spread of sexually transmitted diseases.

Perhaps the greatest health principle given to the Israelites was the invitation to love God supremely, trusting in and depending totally on Him. Disease prevention and long life were promised to all who entered into a relationship with Him. "Worship the Lord your God, and his blessing will be on your food and water. I will take away sickness from among you, and none will miscarry or be barren in your land. I will give you a full life span" (Exodus 23:25, 26, NIV).

Infectious Diseases in the World Today

Infectious diseases have plagued mankind throughout recorded history. Although God gave the Hebrew people various health and sanitation principles, these were largely either unknown or not put into practice by the bulk of humanity. Although industrialized nations have made enormous progress in controlling many of the major infectious diseases, except for smallpox they have not been conquered.

Infectious diseases are caused when a man or woman is made susceptible to a virus, bacteria, or parasite because of various predisposing factors in the environment. To prevent infectious disease, an individual needs to be healthy, receive various immunizations, and have good personal hygiene. The environment needs to be clean, with proper garbage and sewage disposal; control of air, dust, dirt, insects, and animals that may carry the infectious agents; proper handling of food, milk, and water; and isolation of people with severe infectious disease. The infectious agent can be controlled by killing it with heat, cold, radiation, or various chemicals.

Despite our knowledge of these preventive measures, infectious disease remains among the world's major health problems. In the 1970s World Health Organization member states in Asia and Africa were asked to list their most important health problems. Many infectious diseases headed the list, and in order of importance they were malaria and other parasitic diseases, tuberculosis, malnutrition, diarrheal diseases, leprosy, respiratory infections, sexually transmitted diseases, poliomyelitis, and tetanus. In 1984, WHO estimated that in developing countries, infectious diseases that could be prevented by vaccines were responsible for the deaths of some 5 million children per year.

In the United States and other Western nations, the decrease in the number of cases of infectious diseases is the most significant public health success story of the past 100 years. Polio, tetanus, and diphtheria have been virtually eliminated, and although measles, mumps, and pertussis (whooping cough) still cause some problems, the number of children who get these diseases is greatly reduced from what it was just 30 years ago.

Today, two major infectious disease problems that plague people in both developed and developing countries are sexually transmitted diseases (STDs) and infection from the human immunodeficiency virus that leads to acquired immunodeficiency syndrome (AIDS).

STDs are infections spread by transfer of organisms from person to person during sexual contact. More than 50 types of organisms and diseases have now been identified. The most common are gonorrhea, chlamydia, genital warts, genital herpes, and syphilis. More than 12 million cases of STDs occur each year in the United States, 86 percent of them in people aged 15 through 29 years. By age 21 approximately one out of every five young people has required treatment for an STD.

AIDS is the major public health problem of this generation. More than 10 million people worldwide are now believed to be infected with the human immunodeficiency virus (HIV), with two thirds of these cases in Africa, 10 percent in North America, 10 percent in Asia, 9 percent in South and Central America, and 5 percent in Europe. People who are sexually active with multiple partners or who use intravenous drugs are at significant risk for contracting AIDS.

Within several weeks to several months after infection with

HIV, many individuals develop a short-lasting mononucleosis-like illness. Most persons infected with HIV develop antibodies in the blood that can be detected within one to three months, although occasionally there may be a more prolonged interval. HIV-infected persons may then be free of disease symptoms for many months or years before becoming ill. The first phase, called AIDS-related complex, or ARC, starts with a group of symptoms that are not specific. This proceeds to AIDS, which involves more than a dozen different types of unique infections and several cancers.

The proportion of HIV-infected persons who will ultimately develop AIDS is not precisely known. Although the vast majority of HIV-infected persons is projected to develop AIDS within 15 to 20 years, with modern therapy this period is expected to be considerably longer.

Without specific therapy the death rate for AIDS patients has been very high, with 80 to 90 percent of patients dying within three to five years after diagnosis. The HIV attacks the immune system, leaving the person without adequate defense against infectious diseases and cancers.

Regular social or community contact with an HIV-infected person carries no risk of transmission; only sexual contact or exposure to blood or tissues carries a risk. While the HIV has been found in saliva, tears, urine, and lung secretions, there is no evidence that the virus can be transmitted after contact with these secretions.

For both STDs and AIDS, one basic preventive measure is either to not engage in sexual intercourse or to have a mutually faithful sexual relationship with only one uninfected partner.

For HIV infection, the United States Department of Health and Human Services has written that "abstinence from sexual intercourse, monogamous sexual relations with an uninfected partner, and avoidance of intravenous drug use are the most effective means of preventing HIV infection. Proper use of condoms, reducing the number of sexual partners, and abstinence from drug abuse decrease, but do not eliminate, risk of HIV infection'' (*Healthy People 2000: National Health Promotion and Disease Prevention Objectives*, DHHS Pub. No. 91-50212).

Major Chronic or Lifestyle Diseases

The two leading causes of death in the United States and most developed countries around the world are heart disease and cancer. Heart disease is defined as a disease of the heart and its vessels. Most heart disease is caused from blockages in the coronary arteries that supply blood to the heart muscle. Fat and cholesterol, circulating in the blood, are deposited in the inner walls of the arteries. Over the years, scar tissue and other debris build up as more fat and cholesterol are deposited. The arteries become narrower and narrower, much as old water pipes build up layers of mineral deposits. This process is known as atherosclerosis. When one or more of the arteries are seriously narrowed, and then blocked by a blood clot, the result is a heart attack.

In America, 69 million people have one or more forms of heart or blood vessel disease. Nearly 1 million people die every year from heart disease, with 20 percent of these under the age of 65. This represents more than a third of all deaths in the U.S., and costs more than $100 billion per year. Heart disease is our leading killer. (See Table 1.)

From 1920 to 1950 there was a sharp rise in deaths from heart disease, primarily in men. The causes are unknown, but during this time Americans moved off farms into cities, into cars, and increased their dietary intake of meats and dairy products, and began smoking more cigarettes.

In 1953 awareness of the growing epidemic of heart disease increased with the publication of a study of American soldiers killed in action in Korea. Of 300 autopsies on soldiers, average age 22 years, 77 percent of the hearts showed some plaque buildup in the coronary blood vessels.

Since the mid-1960s the sharp rise in deaths from heart disease has been reversed by an equally sharp fall. From 1964 to 1985 heart disease death rates dropped by more than 42 percent, resulting in 350,000 fewer deaths. This decline, impressive for

White men and even steeper in women and Blacks, began in California and spread east. The lowest heart disease death rates are now in the Rocky Mountain states and the highest in the Southeastern states.

Death rates for heart disease have also fallen in Canada, Australia, New Zealand, and Finland, while Eastern Europe has seen marked upturns. However, heart disease is still the major killer of people in developed nations, and much more progress needs to be made.

Table 1   Estimated Total Deaths and Percent of Total Deaths for the 10 Leading Causes of Death: United States, 1987

Rank	Cause of Death	Number	Percent
1	Heart diseases	759,400	35.7
	Coronary heart disease	511,700	24.1
	Other heart disease	247,700	11.6
2	Cancers	476,700	22.4
3	Strokes	148,700	7.0
4	Unintentional injuries	92,500	4.4
5	Chronic obstructive lung diseases	78,000	3.7
6	Pneumonia and influenza	68,600	3.2
7	Diabetes mellitus	37,800	1.8
8	Suicide	29,600	1.4
9	Chronic liver disease and cirrhosis	26,000	1.2
10	Atherosclerosis	23,100	1.1

National Center for Health Statistics, *Monthly Vital Statistics Report*, vol. 37, No. 1, April 25, 1988.

Much has been written about the causes of this dramatic turnaround. Dr. Lee Goldman of Harvard has calculated that approximately 60 percent of the decline in heart disease is related to changes in lifestyle, especially improvements in the diet and a decrease in cigarette smoking. In comparison, about 40 percent of the decline can be attributed to improvements in medical care.

For decades nearly every major health organization in the Western world has been urging people to lower their intake of animal fats and cholesterol, increase intake of plant carbohydrates and fiber, and achieve and maintain a desirable body weight.

In 1988 the surgeon general of the United States submitted a report on nutrition and health, the key statement being: "The report's main conclusion is that overconsumption of certain dietary components is now a major concern for Americans. While many food factors are involved, chief among them is the disproportionate consumption of foods high in fats, often at the expense of foods high in complex carbohydrates and fiber that may be more conducive to health."

Around 1950 Americans began decreasing their intake of eggs, whole milk, butter, and other dairy products. The trend toward a diet lower in animal fats has accelerated recently, as indicated by a comparison of 1977 to 1985 dietary intake. (See Table 2.) These improvements in the American diet have helped to lower serum cholesterol levels and as a result, overall heart disease death rates.

Table 2

Improvement in Diet by Americans (ages 19-50), 1977-1985

Food group	Comparison of food intake between 1977 and 1985	
	Males	Females
Beef	− 35 percent	− 45 percent
Pork	− 7 percent	− 22 percent
Whole milk	− 25 percent	− 35 percent
Eggs	− 26 percent	− 28 percent
Fish	+ 50 percent	+ 18 percent
Low-fat milk	+ 53 percent	+ 60 percent

We now know that several risk factors are associated with heart disease. These factors contribute to an increased risk of heart attack. Table 3 lists the major risk factors. The danger of heart attack increases with the number of risk factors present. Often people who are stricken with heart disease have several risk factors, each of which is only marginally abnormal.

Dr. Jeremiah Stamler, one of America's foremost researchers in the area of health and disease, has estimated that the total effect of eating a low animal fat diet (rather than the typical American diet), having a serum cholesterol of 200 mg./dl. (rather than 240 mg./dl.), a systolic blood pressure of 120 mm. Hg (rather than 140 mm. Hg), and not smoking cigarettes (rather than smoking 10 a day) would add 12 years of life to the average person.

Cancer, in simple terms, is a group of diseases in which abnormal cells grow out of control and can spread throughout the body. Normally, the cells of your body reproduce in an orderly manner so that regular body functions can continue.

Table 3   Risk Factors of Heart Disease

Risk Factors That Cannot Be Changed

• Heredity	Children of parents with heart disease are more likely to develop it themselves.
• Male Sex	Men are at higher risk for heart attacks than women.
• Increasing Age	Older people are at higher risk.

Risk Factors That Can Be Changed

- Cigarette Smoking

This is the most important of all the known risk factors — smokers' risk of heart attack is more than double that of non-smokers. About 50 million Americans are smokers.

- High Blood Pressure

People with blood pressures over 140/90 mm. Hg are at higher risk. More than 60 million Americans have high blood pressure.

- High Blood Cholesterol

The risk of heart disease rises as blood cholesterol levels increase. These should be lower than 200 mg./dl.; levels above 240 mg./dl. more than double the risk. More than 100 million Americans have cholesterol levels above 200 mg./dl.

- Diabetes

Diabetics have a much higher risk of heart disease than others. About 17 million Americans are diabetics; diabetes is most commonly found among overweight people.

- Obesity

People who weigh 20 percent more than they should are at increased risk, especially if much of the fat is in the abdominal area. About 34 million Americans are obese.

- Lack of Exercise

Inactive people have more than double the risk of heart disease compared to the active. Sixty percent of Americans are inactive.

| ● Stress | Excessive amounts of stress over a long time period increase risk of heart disease. Half of U.S. adults report experiencing at least a moderate amount of stress during any given two-week period. |

Adapted from the American Heart Association, *1991 Heart and Stroke Facts*.

Occasionally certain cells undergo an abnormal change and begin a process of uncontrolled growth. These cells may grow into masses of cells called tumors.

In the beginning, cancer cells usually remain at the original site. Later, however, some of the cancer cells may invade neighboring organs or tissues (metastasis). If the cancer is left untreated, it can spread throughout the body, resulting in death. According to the American Cancer Society, about 76 million (or one in three) Americans now living will eventually have cancer. Over the years cancer will strike in approximately three out of four families. More than 20 percent of all deaths in the United States are caused by cancer.

In 1991 more than 1 million people were diagnosed as having cancer, and 514,000 died. Lung cancer is now the leading cancer killer for both men and women, followed by prostate cancer and colon/rectum cancer for men, and breast cancer and colon/rectum cancer for women.

The majority of cancers are now thought to be preventable, with lifestyle and environmental factors related to nearly 90 percent of all cancer cases. The National Cancer Institute estimates that diet is responsible for 35 percent of all cancers, more than any other cause. The estimate for tobacco is 30 percent, with viruses, occupational hazards, alcohol, excess sunshine, and environmental pollution responsible for the rest.

The American Cancer Society has recommended that Americans increase their intake of fruits, vegetables, and whole grains, and decrease their intake of all forms of animal and plant fats to reduce the risk of colon/rectum, prostate, and breast cancers. Obesity should be avoided because it increases risk of colon, breast, prostate, gallbladder, ovary, and uterine cancers. Cigarette smoking, which is responsible for 83 percent of all lung cancers, should be completely avoided. And many oral cancers and cancers of the throat and liver can be prevented by avoiding alcohol consumption.

Why Is Prevention Not Working?

Although we now have knowledge on how to reduce the risk of heart disease, cancer, STDs, and AIDS, this knowledge has not been translated into action by most Americans or effective health and social legislation by the U.S. government to reduce sickness and death.

The three Old Testament principles that we reviewed earlier—proper sanitation, a low animal fat diet, and sexual relations with one faithful life companion—are at the core of modern public health recommendations. And yet from biblical times to now, millions continue to suffer and die from largely preventable diseases.

One major explanation is that apathy exists among many Americans when it comes to living healthfully now for a disease that may happen in the distant future. Whether it is the health crisis or the energy crisis, men and women tend to live for today.

Dr. Ernst Wynder, one of America's foremost preventive medicine advocates, adds that "this public attitude is matched by a similar disinterest among most physicians for preventive measures. Traditionally, physicians are trained to deal with symptoms and find it difficult to adjust their thinking to conditions that have no symptoms. . . . Although many learn by experience, physicians have not been trained in the psychological art of how to motivate people not to smoke, to modify their diets, or to take prescribed medication.

"America's hospitals are not geared to preventive medicine, and the fact that most of our insurance carriers cover principally therapeutic, and not preventive, care compounds the problem.

. . . Physicians must come to regard disease more as a first round that they have lost, as it is reported to have been regarded in China more than 4,000 years ago" (*Journal of the American Medical Association* 229 [1974]: 1743).

Americans are now being urged by many health authorities to rely less on their physicians for health and place more responsibility on themselves. The U.S. Preventive Services Task Force, a group of experts that has submitted guidelines to health professionals for preventive services, recommends that patients assume more responsibility for their health, and that physicians exert more efforts to emphasize lifestyle changes in their counseling to their patients.

In its landmark publication entitled *Guide to Clinical Preventive Services* (Baltimore: Williams and Wilkins, 1989), this task force emphasized that "the most promising role for prevention in current medical practice may lie in changing the personal health behaviors of patients long before clinical disease develops. . . . The increasing evidence of the importance of personal health behaviors and primary prevention means that patients must assume greater responsibility for their own health." It goes on to recommend that all Americans seek to stop smoking, become more active, eat more healthfully, and avoid alcohol and drug abuse, for such actions "hold generally greater promise for improving overall health" than many other clinical activities.

Dr. Bortz writes, "We squander health as we would never squander money. . . . Some people seem to feel that they can walk through a hail of bullets, sail through torpedoes or mine fields, ski down the sides of tall buildings, and somehow land unhurt on their feet. If they are bruised up a bit, well, the docs will fix them up. . . . And still you may protest, 'But what about the patient who drinks like a fish, smokes like a furnace, eats like a hog, carouses like a buck, and is nonetheless 85 years old?' By the same analogy, you may once in a while drive from San Francisco to Los Angeles at 120 miles an hour and still get there—but don't bet on it. Maybe suicide doesn't work the first time around, but try again; the odds get better."

CHAPTER 3

The Adventist
Health Study

*"I saw that it was a sacred duty to attend
to our health."—Ellen G. White, 1863.*

Seventh-day Adventists are among the most researched
groups in the world. Since the 1950s researchers in
Australia, Norway, Japan, Poland, New Zealand, the
Caribbean Islands, the United States, and the Netherlands have
published more than 150 scientific papers on tens of thousands of
Seventh-day Adventists. Why? Because their unique lifestyle has
been associated with dramatic increases in life expectancy and
reductions in death rates from cardiovascular disease and cancer,
the leading killers in Western countries.

The impetus for improving health among Seventh-day Adventists came as a result of a number of visions Ellen G. White
received on health during the mid to late 1800s. Although a major
health reform movement had swept through the United States
beginning in 1830, led on by such reformers as William Alcott,
Sylvester Graham, Horace Fletcher, and John Harvey Kellogg,
most Americans paid little heed.

In the words of Dr. James Whorton, a medical-health
historian, "the large majority of Americans" demonstrated an
inability "to swallow either its bread or doctrine" (*Crusaders for
Fitness* [Princeton, N.J.: Princeton University Press, 1982]).

Through the power and inspiration of Ellen White's visions,

35

however, the Seventh-day Adventist Church embraced essential elements of health practice, and today enjoy the fruits of longer life and lower death rates for most of the major diseases.

In *The Ministry of Healing*, Ellen White describes the cardinal motive behind the health movement within the church. "The knowledge that man is to be a temple for God, a habitation for the revealing of His glory, should be the highest incentive to the care and development of our physical powers. Fearfully and wonderfully has the Creator wrought in the human frame, and He bids us make it our study, understand its needs, and act our part in preserving it from harm and defilement" (p. 271).

In this chapter, you will be brought up to date on the latest research findings regarding the health advantages that many Seventh-day Adventists (SDAs) enjoy.

The Adventist Lifestyle

First a brief summary of the SDA lifestyle. Church policy states that members should abstain completely from tobacco and alcoholic beverages. Since the 1860s the church has highly recommended, but not required, that members practice other health habits such as eating a lacto-ovovegetarian diet (a plant food-based diet that also includes dairy products and eggs), while avoiding coffee and tea, hot condiments and spices, and highly refined foods. A wide variety of fruits, vegetables, whole grains, nuts, and low-fat dairy products are advocated.

SDAs also believe that trust in God, liberal use of pure water, intake of fresh air, moderate exposure to sunlight, participation in daily moderate exercise, and the development of mental capabilities through formal education are important for good health.

SDAs in California have been studied for more than 30 years by researchers at Loma Linda University, and their lifestyle habits have been carefully measured. Although nearly all SDAs in California avoid tobacco and 90 percent report they do not use alcohol, dietary habits vary widely. About 20 percent use meat more than four times per week, compared with 55 percent who follow the lacto-ovovegetarian diet. About 25 percent avoid cheese, while 37 percent use cheese more than three times per week. Close to 30 percent use eggs less than twice a week, while 22 percent use eggs more than five times per week. Seventy-three percent drink less than one cup of coffee per day, with 18 percent drinking more than two cups per day.

Thus California SDAs demonstrate varying degrees of compliance to the health recommendations of the church. This variance is often greater than can be found in the general population, and is one major reason that SDAs have been studied repeatedly. Researchers like to study subgroups of SDAs who differ in lifestyle habits but practice the same religious beliefs, live in the same area, and have similar education and income status. This improves the quality of the research findings.

Increased Life Expectancy

Researchers in various countries have compared life expectancies of SDAs and non-SDAs. Life expectancy refers to the number of years a person can be expected to live at a certain age, usually birth. In California, Norway, Poland, and the Netherlands, SDA males can expect to live from 4.2 to 9.5 years longer than their non-SDA male counterparts, and SDA females 1.9 to 4.6 years longer.

Because not all SDAs follow the lifestyle advocated by their church, these figures are even more impressive when various SDA subgroups are selected. For example, preliminary data suggests that SDA males who follow the complete Adventist lifestyle can expect to live an amazing 12 years longer than non-SDA males.

These are remarkable improvements! Dr. Hans Waaler, who studied SDAs in Norway, explained that "in order for the population in general to achieve the same duration of life, one would have to, for instance, completely eliminate ischemic [blocked coronary arteries that decrease blood and oxygen to the heart muscle] heart disease."

Decrease in Death Rates From Leading Causes

SDAs have been found to live longer because their death rates from both heart disease and cancer are much lower than in non-SDAs throughout the world. SDA men in Japan, Norway, California, and the Netherlands have death rates from heart disease that are approximately half that of non-SDA men. Cancer death rates for SDA men and women combined range from 18 percent to 70 percent less than that of non-SDAs in these same four places.

In a recently published long-term study of 4,342 medical school graduates of Loma Linda University (LLU) (a Seventh-day Adventist university), and 2,832 graduates of the University of Southern California (USC), death rates from heart disease among LLU physicians were reported to be 42 percent lower than among the USC physicians (*Journal of the American Medical Association* 265 [1991]: 2352-2359).

USC physicians were very similar to LLU physicians in many socioeconomic and lifestyle factors (both groups smoked very little). However, USC physicians consumed more meat, eggs, coffee, and alcohol, and less fruit and legumes than the LLU physicians. The LLU physicians also exercised more and smoked less than the USC physicians. This study is considered very important in that it compared two similar groups who ended up differing dramatically in their heart disease death rates because of differing lifestyle habits.

In California, 25,000 SDAs were followed by LLU researchers from 1960 to 1980. From 1977 to 1982, nearly 35,000 California SDAs have been studied in a new phase of the project. From these two study periods, many fascinating results have emerged supporting the importance of a healthy lifestyle in reducing risk of disease and early death.

During the first time period of 1960-1980, 7,250 of the SDAs died, and the causes of death at specific ages were compared with all other United States citizens. SDAs, as expected, were found to have a very low risk of lung cancer and other fatal diseases strongly related to use of cigarettes or alcohol (such as other cancers, heart disease, and stroke). For example, death rates for lung cancer and heart disease are 84 percent and 58 percent lower in SDA men compared to non-SDA men, respectively. SDAs also had lower death rates for diseases unrelated to cigarette and alcohol use such as colon/rectum cancer (50 percent lower), breast cancer (17 percent lower), prostate cancer (26 percent lower), and diabetes (60 percent lower). Amazingly, for all causes of death combined, SDAs were found to have death rates one-half that of the general population. This explains why SDAs live longer. However, they do eventually die of causes similar to those of the general population—they just die at an older age.

Comparison of SDA Subgroups

Some of the most interesting research on SDAs has been comparisons between various SDA subgroups—for example, between SDAs who eat meat and those who do not. With increasing meat use among SDAs, there is a significant increase in risk of dying from heart disease and diabetes, especially in SDA men under the age of 65.

In the age group 45-64 for SDA men, daily use of meat has been associated with a threefold increase in risk of fatal heart disease compared to those who did not eat meat. The lowest risk of fatal heart disease occurred in SDA men and women who practiced the vegetarian diet from an early age (*Preventive Medicine* 13 [1984]: 490-500).

SDAs who weighed 50 percent more than they should had two to four times greater risk of dying from heart disease. SDAs who used more than five eggs a week, drank more than two cups of coffee a day, and weighed 25 percent more than recommended had more colon cancer than lean SDAs who did not drink coffee or used few eggs.

Although use of meat alone was not associated with increased risk of prostate cancer, heavy use of milk, cheese, eggs, and meat in the diet (heavy animal product use) increased risk of fatal prostate cancer threefold. Obesity also increased the risk of fatal prostate cancer in SDAs.

Research findings from the new phase of the Adventist Health Study (1977-1982) are also very interesting. SDAs who ate fruit more than two times a day had a risk for lung cancer 75 percent lower than SDAs who ate fruit less than three times a week (*American Journal of Epidemiology* 133 [1991]: 683-693). High consumption of meat (more than three times a week) by SDAs increased their risk of bladder cancer (*American Journal of Epidemiology* 133 [1991]: 230-239). SDAs consuming higher amounts of vegetarian protein products, beans, lentils, peas, and dried fruit had significantly less pancreas and prostate cancer than SDAs who did not use these foods as much (*Cancer* 61 [1988]: 2578-2585; 64 [1989]: 598-604).

Implications

All of these studies point toward the importance of eating a diet based on cereal grains, legumes, fruits, vegetables, and low-fat dairy products, while avoiding high intakes of saturated fat and cholesterol from meats, whole milk, and high-fat cheeses. This type of diet is now being advocated by nearly every major health and medical organization in the United States.

For instance, in 1988 the surgeon general noted that our nutritional problems today are no longer related to deficiency, but to excess. As the diseases of nutritional deficiency (e.g., scurvy from lack of vitamin C, or pellagra from a lack of niacin) have diminished, they have been replaced by diseases of dietary excess and imbalance. Eight of the top 10 causes of illness and death (in particular, heart disease and cancer) in the United States have been associated with diet and excessive alcohol intake.

While many food factors are involved, the most serious problem of the modern American diet is its high-fat, low-carbohydrate and fiber content. The surgeon general has urged that all Americans reduce the consumption of fat (especially saturated fat) and cholesterol while increasing the intake of carbohydrate and fiber, choosing foods such as vegetables (including dried beans and peas), fruits, whole-grain foods, low-fat dairy products, and for nonvegetarians, low-fat meats. Food preparation methods that add little or no fat are recommended, such as baking or broiling. People are also advised to achieve and maintain a desirable body weight.

Conclusion

SDAs are fortunate to have been pointed in the right direction long before such dietary recommendations became scientifically verified and government-sponsored. SDAs around the world are living longer, and suffering less from heart disease and cancer because they have been advocates of a healthy lifestyle long before it became popular. Basically the Adventist lifestyle boils down to trust in God, daily moderate outdoor exercise, regular and sufficient rest, avoidance of harmful substances, and a healthy lacto-ovovegetarian diet.

It is curious that so many SDAs have not made the decision to fully enter into this lifestyle. While the world eagerly reaches out for all the health and fitness information available, there is some thought that SDAs may be retreating from certain lifestyle practices that have proven to be of such unique advantage.

In chapter 6 we will review the vegetarian diet in more detail, and in chapter 12 the life stories of two very healthy, active elderly SDA women will be upheld as an inspiration to all who may be vacillating on this issue.

CHAPTER 4

The Process of Health Behavior Change

"Choose what is best; habit will soon render it agreeable and easy."—Pythagorus.

M ark Twain once quipped, "Habit is habit, and not to be flung out the window by any man, but coaxed downstairs a step at a time." In this chapter we will review the art and science of health behavior change, one of the greatest challenges many face in their desire for good health and freedom from illness.

America's Poor Health Habits

Americans have much room for health behavior change. *Prevention* magazine, which annually surveys the American public's adherence to 24 important health habits, reports that only one in four Americans practices at least 75 percent of them.

Dr. John Knowles, former director of the Rockefeller Foundation, described it this way: "Americans look upon sloth, gluttony, alcoholic intemperance, reckless driving, sexual frenzy, and smoking as constitutional rights, and they've come to expect government-financed cures for all the unhappy consequences."

Not much has changed from the days of Sylvester Graham, one of America's foremost health reformers, who in the mid-1800s lamented: "It seems as if the grand experiment of mankind has ever been to ascertain how far they can transgress the laws of life; how near they can approach to the very point of death, and yet not die, at least so suddenly and violently, as to be compelled to know that they have destroyed themselves.'' Here are some of the most worrisome details of modern-day American health habits:

● Only 22 percent of Americans exercise appropriately; 60 percent are inactive, with the rest irregular in their habits.

● The average American eats too much fat and too little carbohydrate in the diet. Only 2.5 servings of vegetables and fruits, and three servings of grain products, are consumed daily by the average American, while double this amount is recommended by the National Research Council.

● One out of four Americans is obese, and 75 percent of adults over the age of 40 weigh 10 percent or more than they should.

● Twenty-six percent of Americans smoke cigarettes.

● Alcohol abuse and dependence are serious problems that affect about 10 percent of adult Americans, and are related to more than half of all fatal motor vehicle crashes, homicides, spouse abuse cases, assaults, rapes, manslaughter charges, and drownings.

● Twenty-seven percent of Americans have high blood cholesterol (greater than 240 mg./dl.), and 30 percent have high blood pressure (greater than 140/90 mm. Hg). These conditions are largely the result of improper diet and exercise habits, and being overweight.

• Twenty percent suffer symptoms of sleep deprivation, and 28 percent sleep less than six hours a night.

• One third do not regularly wear their seat belts.

• More than 40 percent of adults report having experienced adverse health effects from stress within the past year.

• About 6 percent of youth aged 12-17 years and 16 percent of young adults aged 18-25 years report having used marijuana during the past month. Cocaine use for these two groups is 1.1 percent and 4.5 percent, respectively.

• The proportion of adolescents who have engaged in sexual intercourse by age 15 is 27 percent for girls and 33 percent for boys. By age 17 these proportions have increased to 50 percent and 66 percent, respectively. Less than one out of five sexually active unmarried women aged 15 through 44 report that their partners used a condom at last sexual intercourse.

• Approximately one third of adolescents report that they have "seriously thought" about committing suicide, and 14 percent report having "actually tried." Ten out of 100,000 adolescents actually commit suicide each year.

• One half to three fourths of all children and adolescents have one or more dental cavities. More than one third of the elderly have lost all their natural teeth.

• Only 21 percent of mothers are still breast-feeding their babies at 5 to 6 months. Twenty-five percent of pregnant mothers smoke during pregnancy.

Do Good Health Habits Really Help?

Adopting good health habits does result in meaningful improvements in health and longevity. One of the best studies was done by Dr. Lester Breslow of the University of California, Los Angeles. He studied the personal health habits of 7,000 adults in the San Francisco Bay area and showed a strong relationship between seven simple health habits and their physical health status. Reports Dr. Breslow, "The physical health status of those following all seven good health practices was consistently about the same as those 30 years younger who followed few or none of these practices" (*Preventive Medicine* 9 [1980]: 469-483).

What were the seven health habits Dr. Breslow used in his study? They are some very basic health habits that many mothers have been bidding family members to practice for generations—seven to eight hours of sleep regularly, maintaining proper weight, eating breakfast, not eating between meals, never smoking cigarettes, moderate or no use of alcohol, and regular physical activity. The results of this study agree with the recent pronouncement of the U.S. surgeon general that two thirds of the ailments encountered before age 65 are preventable.

Obviously the most important challenge for the future is helping Americans to practice healthful personal behaviors. Much work is to be done, and all are invited to participate in the process.

The Process of Health Behavior Change

"Habit is a cable; we weave a thread of it every day, and at last we cannot break it" (Horace Mann).

How do you go about starting a regular exercise program, or becoming a vegetarian, or losing excess body weight, or quitting smoking? Scientists have studied this issue in much detail, and have come up with three basic principles to guide people as they seek to change their behavior.

First, accurate health information is necessary but not sufficient to cause people to change their health behavior. In other words, knowing that exercise is important to health is one thing, doing it is another. There are many nonexercising physical educators, obese cardiologists, junk food-eating nutritionists, smoking doctors, and cocaine-using counselors.

Second, if people perceive that they are susceptible to acquiring a certain grievous disease (e.g., cancer) because of their lifestyle (e.g., smoking), and understand both the benefits and barriers involved in changing their behavior, and are convicted about their ability to carry out the recommended action (quitting smoking), health behavior change is more likely.

Finally, many personal, environmental, cultural, family, and group factors exist that influence the likelihood of health behavior change. Individuals who have a purpose in life and long-term goals; are open and receptive to others; have strong social ties; possess an optimistic and hopeful attitude and a positive self-image; have a supportive spouse and family and a favorable economic status; and retain employer and coworker support are much more likely to improve their health behavior when given the chance than others.

The process of health behavior change has several steps:

Step 1—Preparation. An individual becomes educated about certain health behaviors. He or she is instructed on how to go about carrying out the behavior, and develops commitment to the idea while developing reasonable expectations of what can be expected.

This step demands the cooperation of health professionals such as medical doctors, health educators, and other health workers who have the appropriate training and information, and know how to deliver it in a motivating fashion.

Often it is helpful to be screened or tested for certain risk factors (blood pressure, serum cholesterol, percent body fat, lung function, nutrient intake, physical fitness, etc.). The testing process can be a real eye-opener for some people who are in self-denial about their health status.

Step 2—Goal Setting and Contracting. With help from the health professional, family, and friends, goals are set that are adapted to the person's unique circumstances. An actual contract should be written in very specific terms. However, the goals, while very specific, should be flexible, and changed periodically if necessary. For example, a goal to walk two to three miles a day from 5:15 to 6:00 p.m. for two months straight may be established. However, if after a week this seems unrealistic, the duration or the time of day can be changed in the contract.

Step 3—Shaping. Health behaviors are best changed or shaped gradually, usually one by one, with a conservative start to ensure success. Changing many behaviors at once usually leads to failure and disappointment. That in turn leads to disbelief in the whole idea. For example, if an overweight smoker decides to improve his health, the first goal would be to quit smoking, and then later to work on his body weight, both under two separate contract arrangements.

Step 4—Reinforcement. When certain goals are met at designated times (e.g., to quit smoking or lose weight), rewards from family members or colleagues should be arranged and stipulated in the contract. The rewards can be anything of meaning to the individual who is changing the health behavior. For example, if a woman meets a goal of losing 10 pounds in six weeks and then maintaining the loss for another four weeks, the reward may be a new dress or a weekend vacation.

Step 5—Stimulus Control. This means setting up a system of cues or reminders at home and work to encourage adherence to the new health behavior until it becomes more habitual. A good idea is to write down the actual health behavior in the appropriate time slot in your schedule. Keep it posted in areas where you are throughout the day. Alarms or notes from family members can also be used as reminders.

Step 6—Cognitive Strategies. A balance sheet of advantages and disadvantages involved in the health behavior change can be drawn up and reviewed from time to time to reinforce continued adherence. The person should focus on the increased feelings of health, self-esteem, and enjoyment being experienced.

Step 7—Social Support. The support of one's spouse, family members, coworkers, and friends is critical, and should be organized by someone close to the individual who is seeking change in some behavior. For example, if an individual is trying to stop smoking, an organized network of support can be arranged by the spouse to give him encouragement.

Step 8—Relapse Prevention. The individual should prepare for some occasions of failure, and have ways to cope when they happen. These situations can be anticipated, and either avoided, modified, or dealt with with the help of others. Relapse should be viewed not as a failure but a challenge to carry on.

Cooperation With God

For the Christian, there is the added bonus of divine support and power. The Bible presents the viewpoint that although mankind is weak, God is almighty and powerful, and as we unite our faltering efforts with His strength, His way becomes our desire, as the Holy Spirit helps us with our daily challenges (Romans 8:26, 27; John 3:5). Paul described it this way: "To this end I labor, struggling with all his energy, which so powerfully works in me" (Colossians 1:29, NIV).

Our motive for change, Paul reminds us, is God's love and mercy. "Therefore, I urge you, brothers, in view of God's mercy, to offer your bodies as living sacrifices, holy and pleasing to God—this is your spiritual act of worship" (Romans 12:1, NIV). John adds, "How great is the love the Father has lavished on us, that we should be called children of God! And that is what we are! . . .

"Everyone who has this hope in him purifies himself, just as he is pure" (1 John 3:1-3, NIV). In other words, we seek health behavior change, not to earn acceptance from God or salvation, but because "Christ's love compels us" (2 Corinthians 5:14, NIV).

When this motive governs our decisions and actions, the Scriptures portray a change process that is "not burdensome" (1 John 5:3). Christ pointed out that "my yoke is easy and my burden is light" (Matthew 11:30, NIV), while the psalmist relates that God's will becomes our desire (Psalm 40:8). God is not in the business of burdening us; instead, He has repeatedly reminded us that He will carry our burdens (Deuteronomy 30:11-14; Micah 6:3; Psalm 55:22; 68:19; Isaiah 43:23, 24).

As the change in health behavior takes place, and the fruitage of improved health is experienced, we can give God full praise, for He is the source of the power for change. "I can do everything through him who gives me strength" (Philippians 4:13, NIV). "For from him and through him and to him are all things. To him be the glory forever!" (Romans 11:36, NIV).

CHAPTER 5

Exercising
Your Right to Health

*"In the curse pronounced upon our first parents
there is annexed a peculiar blessing, a circumstance
so strikingly characteristic of Deity. It was
pronounced upon Adam, 'In the sweat of thy brow
shalt thou earn thy bread.' In the very sweat
produced by labor or exercise the blessing of
health is found, which may be sought for in vain
from any other source."—Woster Beach, 1857.*

Mark Twain once described the health fanatic as one "who eats what he doesn't want, drinks what he doesn't like, and does what he'd druther not, all the while smugly announcing himself to be energetic, joyful, and certain of long life, and exhorting his errant neighbor to reform." Along the same lines, Oliver Wendell Holmes once snickered, "Some men seem to 'seek to merit heaven by making earth a hell,' and we can readily conceive how a dyspeptic in his closet might look a little enviously upon his sleek and oily neighbor, who sleeps well, eats well, and perchance smokes his cigar."

The healthy lifestyle has often been viewed as a long list of things *not* to do. The modern-day fitness movement has helped to change this image. Regular exercise is a positive addition to the lifestyle, something good to do. Even more than this, there is some evidence that the decision to start an exercise program often leads to many other healthy changes.

Dr. Roy Shephard from the University of Toronto, Ontario, Canada, has been a leading advocate of the concept that exercise can lead to other desirable health behaviors such as a low-fat diet, while helping a person eliminate undesirable habits such as cigarette smoking. Likewise, moderate outdoor exercise, such as walking, increases the intake of fresh air into the lungs while at the same time it brings a dose of sunshine.

Dr. Shephard feels that research "evidence links regular exercise and/or personal fitness with various favorable health behaviors," and that "exercise is also tied to many perceived health benefits."

Regular exercise also leads to many direct health advantages. In this chapter we will review the results of studies worldwide that have documented the benefits of exercise, confirming the wisdom of Socrates who long ago proposed, "And is not bodily habit spoiled by rest and illness, but preserved for a long time by motion and exercise?"

Designed to Move

There is a God-given design in nature for action and movement. Consider the flowers that open and close daily or the circulating ocean currents and orbiting planets. Water is fresh and clean if taken from a rushing stream, but unhealthful when drawn from a stagnant pond.

God especially stamped the law of action in mankind, and it is inherent in every particle of his being. Ellen White has written, "Action is a law of our being. Every organ of the body has its appointed work, upon the performance of which its development and strength depend. The normal action of all the organs gives strength and vigor, while the tendency of disuse is toward decay and death" (*The Ministry of Healing*, p. 237).

Physical work was provided by God from the beginning. "The Lord God took the man and put him in the Garden of Eden to work it and take care of it" (Genesis 2:15, NIV). And upon the introduction of sin, the intensity of effort required was increased. " 'Cursed is the ground because of you; through painful toil you will eat of it all the days of your life. It will produce thorns and thistles for you, and you will eat the plants of the field. By the sweat of your brow you will eat your food' '' (Genesis 3:17-19, NIV). But as was noted in the quote by Woster Beach at the beginning of this chapter, with the hard physical labor came ''the blessing of health'' as man fulfilled the design of his body.

Four chief benefits are associated with exercise: improvement in heart and lung function, increase in psychological well-being, prevention of disease, and retardation of the aging process. Before reviewing these, lets consider what most fitness experts are now recommending regarding the quantity and type of exercise needed to produce these benefits.

The American College of Sports Medicine, the foremost authorative organization in the world on exercise, recommends that for both health and fitness, people should exercise at moderate intensities for 30 to 60 minutes daily. These new guidelines are different from earlier positions published by the American College of Sports Medicine, in which they recommended more vigorous levels of exercise for shorter periods of time.

Several national surveys have shown that the majority of Americans who do exercise regularly use walking as their major form of activity. Fitness leaders agree that brisk walking is most appropriate because it includes the major benefits of exercise without some of the harmful risks that come with higher intensity activities such as running.

Dr. James Rippe of the University of Massachusetts, one of America's leading authorities on walking, has written, ''In the past decade a quiet revolution has taken place in the way Americans think and act about exercise. . . . Walking has emerged as a particularly appealing activity to promote health and fitness. . . . Walking provides an effective form of activity to help people establish the kind of consistent, lifelong exercise programs that have been shown to carry the most important long-term health benefits'' (*Journal of the American Medical Association* 259 [1988]: 2720-2724).

Thomas Jefferson once declared, ''The sovereign invigorator of the body is exercise, and of all exercises walking is the best.''

Ellen White expressed the same conviction. "A walk, even in winter, would be more beneficial to the health than all the medicine the doctors may prescribe." "There is no exercise that can take the place of walking. By it the circulation of the blood is greatly improved" (*Counsels on Health*, pp. 52, 200).

Improvement in Heart and Lung Function

"Even youths grow tired and weary, and young men stumble and fall; but those who hope in the Lord will renew their strength. They will soar on wings like eagles; they will run and not grow weary, they will walk and not be faint" (Isaiah 40:30, 31, NIV).

Let's say that as you are reading this chapter, you suddenly notice black smoke rising from your friend's apartment complex, which is one mile away. If you were to run to your friend's aid, you would notice several immediate changes in body function. Your breathing rate would quicken as you take in larger quantities of air with each breath, supplying more vital oxygen to your body. You might observe that your heart is pounding faster as it pumps more blood to your active leg muscles. If your pace is too quick, you may feel a burning sensation in your legs as the lactic acid concentration increases. These sudden, temporary changes in body function caused by exercise are called acute responses to exercise and disappear shortly after the exercise period is finished.

If you were to exercise briskly every day, after a few weeks you might see some changes in the way your body functions during both rest and exercise. You might notice that your heart beats slower while you sit and study, and also during your exercise. The amount of air you breathe in during a certain type of exercise might decrease, and you might feel less of a burning sensation in your legs.

These persistent changes in the structure and function of your body following regular exercise training are called chronic adaptations to exercise. These adjustments apparently enable the body to respond more easily to subsequent exercise bouts.

The key element in exercise is the amount of oxygen you take in. Oxygen is needed to burn body fuels, supplying the energy needed for muscular movement. As you become physically fit, many changes occur in the body to ensure more oxygen to the working muscles. The most important change is an increase in the size of the heart, which allows more blood to be pumped with each beat. The heart becomes a more efficient pump, which leads to a decrease in both your resting and exercise heart rates. It is common for people to lower their resting heart rates 10 to 20 beats per minute after three to four months of regular exercise.

The lungs can take in more air and deliver more oxygen to the blood after a period of exercise training. The amount of blood in the body increases, and more blood vessels grow in the areas of the body used during the exercise bouts. The muscles build up their supply of both fuel and enzymes to burn the fuel.

The net result of all these changes is that oxygen can be taken from the air you breathe much easier, and then delivered by the heart and blood to the working muscles in a much more efficient manner. You have become physically fit and can walk up stairs or carry loads of groceries much easier than before.

Interestingly, these improvements happen rather quickly (within several weeks), but can be lost just as easily. The body is designed to exercise daily, and only through regular exercise can the heart and lungs stay fit.

Increase in Psychological Well-being

"A turn or two I'll walk, to still my beating mind" (Shakespeare).

"In walking, the will and the muscles are so accustomed to working together and perform their task with so little expenditure of force that the intellect is left comparatively free" (Oliver Wendell Holmes).

We are devoting a portion of chapter 10 to the discussion of this unique benefit of exercise. Most people who exercise regularly claim that their main reason for doing so is "to feel better." A large number of studies have now been published showing that anxiety, depression, and mental stress can be decreased with exercise, while feelings of general well-being, short-term ability to think, and self-concept are improved. We will review this evidence in detail in chapter 11.

Prevention of Disease

"Anyone who lives a sedentary life and does not exercise— even if he eats good foods and takes care of himself according to proper medical principles—all his days will be painful ones and his strength shall wane" (Maimonides).

"Every man has two doctors, his right leg and his left" (ancient proverb).

As we have discussed earlier in this book, heart disease and cancer are the two leading killers in the United States today. We now have good evidence that regular exercise can help decrease the risk of both.

People who are physically active tend to weigh less, have lower blood pressure and serum cholesterol levels, and as a result, are at a much lower risk for heart disease than their inactive counterparts.

The Centers for Disease Control (CDC) reviewed 43 of the major studies worldwide that have been conducted on exercise and heart disease. They concluded that the risk for heart disease in sedentary people is double that of the physically active, and that this is the same degree of risk involved for those who smoke or have high blood pressure or serum cholesterol levels.

The CDC researchers summarized their review by writing, "In general, these studies show that both physical fitness and physical activity (whether on the job or during leisure) are associated with decreased risk of heart disease, and that regular physical activity should be promoted as vigorously as blood pressure control, dietary modification to lower serum cholesterol, and smoking cessation" (*Annual Reviews of Public Health* 8 [1987]: 253-287). Researchers go on to explain that the percentage of Americans who are inactive is much greater than for the other heart disease risk factors. (See Table 1.) Because so many people are inactive, unusual efforts should be made to promote physical activity in this country.

Table 1

A Comparison of the Prevalence of Several Major Risk Factors for Coronary Heart Disease

Risk Factor	Percent of U.S. Population
Cigarette smoking	30
High serum cholesterol levels	25
High blood pressure	30
Obesity	25
Inactivity	60
Irregular activity	33
Completely sedentary	27

How much physical exercise is needed to prevent heart disease? At the Institute for Aerobics Research in Dallas, Texas, Dr. Stephen Blair studied more than 13,000 men and women for eight years. Heart disease death rates were eight times greater in the "poor" aerobic fitness group compared to the "good" fitness group. Cancer death rates were also several times higher in the "poor" aerobic fitness group. Dr. Blair concluded that avoidance of "poor" fitness is paramount, "which can be accomplished by 30-60 minutes of brisk walking each day" (*Journal of the American Medical Association* 262 [1989]: 2395-2401).

Regarding cancer, several researchers have shown that people in sedentary jobs have a 30-100 percent greater risk of getting colon cancer than people with more active jobs. Active women have been found to experience less breast and uterine cancers.

Some researchers have theorized that moderate exercise stimulates muscle movement (peristalsis) of the large intestine, shortening the time that the colon wall is in contact with any cancer causing chemicals in the fecal matter. In other words, regular moderate exercise is like dietary fiber—both help food contents to get through the colon faster, reducing cancer risk.

The important lesson from all of the research we have reviewed in this section is that heart disease and cancer risk are greatest in people who do virtually no exercise. Protection from these diseases develops when just 30 to 60 minutes of moderate exercise, like walking, is engaged in regularly.

Retardation of the Aging Process

"Much of the human deterioration that we attribute to aging is simply a manifestation of deconditioning caused by inactivity" (Dr. Lawrence Morehouse).

"Walking makes for a long life" (Hindu proverb).

In chapter 12 we will have much more to say on this exciting benefit of exercise. As a person ages, heart and lung function decrease by about 1 percent a year after 25 years of age. However, half of this decline is probably occurring because people tend to exercise less as they grow older.

Is it possible for elderly people to forestall the decrease in heart and lung function through regular exercise? In chapter 11 we will review the test results of two remarkable women, Mavis Lindgren and Hulda Crooks, who, despite being 85 and 95, respectively (in 1992), have the heart and lungs of much younger women because of their exercise programs.

Many researchers have now shown that men and women in their 60s and 70s are able, through exercise, to increase their heart and lung function above that of healthy but inactive young adults in their 20s and 30s.

Can you live longer if you exercise? Dr. Ralph Paffenbarger of Stanford University showed that Harvard University alumni who exercised regularly could expect to live 2.2 years longer than inactive alumni. Dr. Paffenbarger emphasized that "this has the same statistical impact of removing cancer from the United States. . . . This improvement in longevity can be gained by walking or jogging 8-10 miles a week'' (*New England Journal of Medicine* 314 [1986]: 605-613).

Concluding Remarks

Shakespeare in *Hamlet* wrote, ''What a piece of work is a man! how noble in reason! how infinite in faculty!'' When we perceive the fact that we truly are wonderfully made by our Creator God, that regular exercise is a matter of function meeting design, and that major benefits occur with just 30 to 60 minutes of daily moderate activity, taking time out of a busy schedule may be just a bit easier.

CHAPTER 6

A Diet for
All Time

"Not so the Golden Age, that fed on fruit,
Nor durst with bloody meats their mouth pollute.
Then birds in airy space might safely move,
And timorous hares on heaths securely rove;
Nor needed fish the guileful hooks to fear,
For all was peaceful, and that peace sincere."—Ovid.

Interest in a vegetarian diet is at an all-time high. One of the most significant reasons is the large number of government-sponsored diet-health reports that have urged Americans to eat less meat and dairy products, and more whole grains, fruits, and vegetables. At the same time, researchers worldwide have published reports on the many health and fitness benefits in those who practice the vegetarian lifestyle.

In this chapter we will review the history of vegetarianism, and both the scientific and biblical grounds for this kind of diet. Before we look at the evidence, let's define some terms.

There are several types of vegetarians, and it is easy to become confused. Vegetarians differ as to the extent they avoid animal products, restrict other foods and beverages, and use special foods or supplements thought to have unique health or medical benefits.

A vegetarian is generally defined as a person who lives wholly or principally on plant foods, abstaining from meat. A total vegetarian, or vegan, avoids animal foods of all kinds, including eggs and dairy products.

The lacto-vegetarian consumes milk or milk products, but no

eggs. The lacto-ovovegetarian includes dairy products and eggs in the diet. Most Seventh-day Adventists who are vegetarian are lacto-ovovegetarians. Few Adventists are vegan.

Semivegetarians consume some animal flesh. Usually they will avoid red meat, like beef and pork, but will use poultry and seafood. Fruitarians use fruit as the staple in their diet, avoiding to a large extent all other types of foods. This is a dangerous diet in that many nutrients are lacking.

New vegetarians tend to be people who are attracted to the vegetarian lifestyle but are somewhat restrictive in the types of plant foods they eat. Often new vegetarians have inadequate nutrition knowledge to make wise food choices, and as a result may become malnourished.

Reasons people give for being vegetarian can be grouped in these general categories: (1) spiritual; (2) health and disease prevention; (3) nutrition; (4) economic and ecological; (5) ethical; (6) fitness.

Spiritual

"I am conscious that flesh eating is not in accordance with the finer feelings" (Albert Schweitzer).

Some vegetarians give statements from the Bible as their major reason for avoiding the consumption of meat. They point out that in the Garden of Eden, where no killing took place, God provided plant foods for Adam and Eve to eat. "Then God said, 'I give you every seed-bearing plant on the face of the whole earth and every tree that has fruit with seed in it. They will be yours for food'" (Genesis 1:29, NIV).

In addition, God provided the Israelites with manna in the desert, and gave them meat only when they clamored for it (Exodus 16:14-35; Numbers 11:4-34). Such Bible heroes as Daniel and John the Baptist are upheld for their avoidance of meat (Daniel 1:8-16; Matthew 3:4). And Isaiah points out that on the earth made new, "the wolf and the lamb will feed together, and the lion will eat straw like the ox. . . . They will neither harm nor destroy on all my holy mountain" (Isaiah 65:25, NIV).

On the other hand, there are instances in the Bible when meat is eaten. For example, Jesus is reported to have eaten meat (Luke 22:7, 8, 15; 24:42, 43). God gave permission for mankind to eat meat after the flood (Genesis 9:3) and to the Hebrews after their desert wanderings (Deuteronomy 12:15, 16, 20).

Abraham prepared meat for his heavenly guests (Genesis 18:8), as did Gideon (Judges 6:19), and ravens from the Lord brought Elijah bread and flesh each morning and evening (1 Kings 17:6). Several of the sacrificial ceremonies of the Hebrews involved the eating of flesh (Exodus 12:8; Leviticus 7:15; 8:31).

The early Christians ate meat and argued long and hard about whether they should eat flesh if it had been offered to pagan idols (Acts 15:20; 1 Corinthians 8; Romans 14).

However, some vegetarians argue that the consumption of meat in the Bible reflects God's concessions to less than ideal conditions.

Dr. James Whorton, a medical-health historian from the University of Washington in Seattle, has reviewed the early history of vegetarianism in the United States, and the close ties of this movement to religion (*Crusaders for Fitness*).

The essential creed of health reform during the 1800s, states Whorton, was the belief "that the Kingdom of Health, like the Kingdom of Heaven, is within you" and was to be gained by hygienic righteousness.

In his chapter entitled "Tempest in a Flesh-Pot," Whorton summarizes the activities of health reformers such as Sylvester Graham and those in the American Vegetarian Society, founded in 1850, who mixed science and religion to promote their views.

Concerns of the health reformers during this period were twofold: that the killing and eating of animals "contaminated and brutalized the human soul," and that health and fitness were superior in vegetarians. Spirited verbal battles between vegetarian health reformers and other scientists who advocated a meat-based diet continued until the turn of the century.

In 1863, after her first major vision on health, Ellen White began promoting the vegetarian diet for the Seventh-day Adventist church. In the chapter entitled "Flesh as Food" in *The*

Ministry of Healing, Mrs. White writes, "The diet appointed man in the beginning did not include animal food. . . . In choosing man's food in Eden, the Lord showed what was the best diet. . . . Flesh was never the best food; but its use is now doubly objectionable, since disease in animals is so rapidly increasing. . . . The moral evils of a flesh diet are not less marked than are the physical ills. Flesh food is injurious to health, and whatever affects the body has a corresponding effect on the mind and the soul" (pp. 311-315).

Many Seventh-day Adventists took the challenge to change their diets, and today an estimated half are vegetarian, making them the largest group of "traditional" vegetarians in the United States. As we'll see in the next section, this has led to many health benefits.

Health and Disease Prevention

"A considerable body of scientific data suggests positive relationships between vegetarian lifestyles and risk reduction for several chronic degenerative diseases, such as obesity, coronary artery disease, hypertension, diabetes mellitus, colon cancer, and others" (American Dietetic Association, 1988).

The American Dietetic Association published this statement in its position paper on the vegetarian diet (*Journal of the American Dietetic Association* 88 [1988]: 352-355). Much of the support for the connection between vegetarianism and disease prevention comes from the Adventist Health Study by Loma Linda University, research that has been ongoing since 1960.

In chapter 3 of this book, we reviewed some of the major findings from this study. Results show that vegetarian SDAs have considerably less heart disease, cancer, and diabetes than non-vegetarians. While some of this is related to the avoidance of tobacco and alcohol, evidence is mounting that restriction of meat, along with the high consumption of plant foods, also plays a major role.

For example, SDAs who eat meat have a much higher risk of heart disease than SDAs who are vegetarian. And SDAs who became vegetarian at an early age have the best protection from heart disease. Adventists who eat high amounts of fruits and vegetables have lower rates of cancer than do Adventists or non-Adventists who eat few.

Similar results have been found in other vegetarian groups in the United States, Germany, England, Australia, and China. Dr. Colin Campbell of Cornell University has been studying more than 6,000 people in China since 1983, and has concluded that their diet of primarily rice and vegetables is protecting them from many of the diseases that plague Western men and women.

Dr. Walter Willett of Harvard University followed 89,000 women for six years and concluded "that a higher consumption of red meat and fat from animal sources increases the incidence of colon cancer" (*New England Journal of Medicine* 323 [1990]: 1664-1672). In San Francisco, Dr. Dean Ornish reported that the combination of a low-fat vegetarian diet, smoking cessation, stress management, and moderate exercise actually reversed atherosclerosis (plaque buildup in the coronary heart vessels) in 82 percent of his patients (*Lancet* 336 [1990]: 129-133).

Why does a vegetarian diet help prevent heart disease and cancer? Regarding cancer, most researchers feel that the high-fiber, low-fat nature of the vegetarian diet as a whole, and various substances found in fruits and vegetables (e.g., beta-carotene, trace minerals, and special chemicals called "phytochemicals"), have a protective effect against many kinds of cancers. Several studies have shown that the vegetarian diet changes blood hormone levels and decreases certain cancer-causing chemicals in the colon, lowering risk of cancer.

With regard to heart disease, because a plant-based diet has no cholesterol, is low in saturated fat, and high in dietary fiber, blood cholesterol levels and blood pressure tend to be much lower in vegetarians than in meat eaters. In one study, for example, SDA vegans had a serum cholesterol level of 149 mg./dl. compared to 214 mg./dl. for a group of non-SDA meat eaters (*American Journal of Clinical Nutrition* 40 [1984]: 921-926).

Other vegetarians around the world have also been measured to have very low serum cholesterol levels. In northern Mexico, the Tarahumara Indians, who eat primarily corn, beans, and some greens, have an average serum cholesterol level of 136 mg./dl. In rural China, where people eat three times more fiber and less than half the fat of Americans, serum cholesterol levels range from 90 to 175 mg./dl., which is at the lowest end of the American range.

Vegetarians also tend to weigh less than meat eaters, which helps prevent heart disease, cancer, and diabetes. In a study by Dr. Mervyn Hardinge of Loma Linda University, SDA vegan males and females weighed 146 and 117 pounds, respectively, compared to 170 and 142 pounds, respectively, for meat eaters.

Is there any special advantage to eating a vegetarian diet compared to a low-fat meat diet? In other words, most health groups today advocate that Americans increase their intake of plant foods and low-fat meats and dairy products, while avoiding fatty animal foods. Is this adequate?

In a study done by a team of researchers in Australia, the lacto-ovovegetarian diet was compared with a low-fat meat-based diet and a high-fat meat-based diet. Subjects in the low-fat meat diet ate one-half pound of lean meat a day, while the vegetarians ate meat substitutes made from wheat gluten and soybeans. After six weeks on the various diets, the vegetarian diet ended up decreasing the serum cholesterol twice as much as did the low-fat meat diet (compared to the high-fat meat diet). The researchers concluded that the vegetarian diet "conferred the greater benefit" (*Ibid*, 50 [1989]: 280-287).

Safety Concerns About Meat

Each year millions of cases of food-borne illness occur from a wide variety of bacteria that are in many foods, primarily meat, eggs, and dairy products. The Centers for Disease Control reported 9,000 deaths in 1983 from such food poisoning, which usually causes people to be sick for one to 10 days. Most outbreaks occur because people do not store, prepare, cook, or serve the food properly. Fruits and vegetables rarely cause problems.

Poultry is the food most often contaminated with disease-causing organisms. It's estimated by the Food and Drug Administration that 60 percent or more of raw poultry sold at retail probably carries some disease-causing bacteria (*FDA Consumer*, January-February 1991). Various bacteria have been found in raw seafood. Also, oysters, clams, mussels, scallops, and cockles may be carriers of hepatitis A virus. Fish and shellfish are responsible for about one in four food-borne illnesses, and most of the cases result from seafood taken from contaminated and polluted water.

While most food-borne illnesses can be prevented by avoidance of raw seafood or by thorough cooking and proper storage, recent concern has been raised over the use of antibiotics and hormones in animal feed. All turkeys, 80 percent of swine, 80 percent of veal calves, 60 percent of cattle, and 30 percent of chickens are raised on antibiotic-laced feed, according to the U.S. Food and Drug Administration. Antibiotics are used to prevent infection in these animals and promote their growth. These drugs have been used for more than 30 years now, and farm animals devour more than 15 million pounds of antibiotics each year.

This massive use of antibiotics on the farm is breeding strains of drug-resistant microorganisms. Several research studies indicate that commercially produced animal meats may be a path by which resistant bacteria reach humans, causing food poisoning that is hard to treat with antibiotics (*Journal of the American Medical Association* 258 [1987]: 1496-1499).

More research is needed to confirm these concerns, but it is now calculated that many of the cases of food poisoning each year are caused by bacteria in meat and poultry products from animals given antibiotic-laced feed. This increases the danger that our lifesaving antibiotics may become less and less effective. The Food and Drug Administration is seeking to restrict the use of antibiotics in animal feed.

Obviously one way to reduce risk of food poisoning is to be a vegan. Lacto-ovovegetarians are also at reduced risk, especially if they are particularly careful when handling eggs.

Regarding milk, a two-month FDA study of 70 milk samples from 14 cities showed virtually no presence of antibiotic drug residues. The FDA report suggests that only a few animals whose milk is being sold are improperly treated with drugs (*FDA Consumer*, July-August 1990). However, the Center for Science in the Public Interest claims that the FDA underestimated the seriousness of the problem of drug residues in milk, and that further study is needed.

Recently the Food and Drug Administration allowed dairy farmers to sell milk from cows injected with bovine growth hormone, also known as bovine somatotropin, or bST. This hormone allows the cow to increase its milk production. While many consumer groups and dairy farmers feel that milk from these cows is unsafe, the FDA and the National Institutes of Health have both come down on the side of research indicating complete safety.

The FDA has stated that "milk and meat from bST-supplemented experimental dairy cows may be used for human consumption without causing a risk to the public health" (*ibid*, April 1990). The National Institutes of Health has concluded that the "composition and nutritional value of milk from bST-treated cows is essentially the same as that of milk from untreated cows. As currently used in the United States, meat and milk from bST-treated cows are as safe as that from untreated cows" (*Journal of the American Medical Association* 265 [1991]: 1423-1425).

What about the risk of pesticide residues on fruits, vegetables, and grains to the health of people like vegetarians who eat large quantities of plant foods? It is estimated that pests destroy about a third of the world's food crops every year. To control these pests, in the United States alone, 1.6 billion pounds of pesticides are used per year.

Although there is some reason to be less than comfortable

about the kinds and amounts of pesticides allowed on foods, the risk to consumers appears to be very small (*Nutrition Today*, November/December 1989).

The FDA conducts a comprehensive monitoring program that measures pesticide residues in foods. In 1987 no legal tolerance violations of pesticide residues were found in more than 95 percent of the 14,000 marketplace samples the FDA analyzed. In 1988 more than 96 percent of the 18,000 samples of fruits, vegetables, and grain products analyzed by the FDA either contained no residues of pesticides or the levels found were well below legally permitted limits (*FDA Consumer*, March 1990).

Nutritional

"Grains, fruits, nuts, and vegetables constitute the diet chosen for us by our Creator. These foods, prepared in as simple and natural a manner as possible, are the most healthful and nourishing "(Ellen G. White).

The American Dietetic Association has now affirmed that a well-planned diet consisting of a variety of plant products (unrefined), supplemented with some milk and eggs (lacto-ovovegetarian), meets all known nutrient needs. Even a total plant food diet (no meat, eggs, or dairy products) can be nutritionally adequate with proper food planning.

In fact, the American Dietetic Association has gone on record stating that "it may be easier, as well as more acceptable, for some individuals to meet the Dietary Guidelines for Americans by following a vegetarian diet rather than a nonvegetarian diet" (*Journal of the American Dietetic Association* 88 [1988]: 351).

Any individual, but especially infants, children, and pregnant and lactating women, can be at risk if the vegan or total vegetarian diet is not well planned.

In planning a vegetarian diet, choose a wide variety of foods from the major food groups. The foods may include fresh fruits, vegetables, whole grain breads and cereals, nuts and seeds, legumes, low-fat dairy products, meat substitutes, such as gluten or soybean products, and a limited number of eggs, if desired.

Vegans who avoid all animal products must ensure that they eat enough to maintain desirable body weight, especially during childhood. This is best accomplished by eating more nuts, dried fruits, legumes, and grain products.

Vegans must also be certain to include an appropriate source of vitamin B_{12} in their diets because this vitamin is not found in any plant food.

In one study of 150 people eating the macrobiotic diet, a vegan diet that typically consists of 50-60 percent whole cereal grains, 20-25 percent vegetables, and 5-10 percent beans and sea vegetables, the majority were found to have low serum vitamin B_{12} levels, especially in the strict vegans (*American Journal of Clinical Nutrition* 53 [1991]: 524-529). Vitamin B_{12} can be provided as a supplement to the vegan diet, or come from fortified foods such as breakfast cereals or soymilk.

If a vegan's exposure to sunshine is limited, a vitamin D supplement may be needed. Most people get enough of this vitamin when they drink vitamin D-fortified milk. In one study of 53 infants on a macrobiotic diet, physical symptoms of rickets were present in 28 percent of the babies during the summer and 55 percent of them during the winter. The researchers concluded that the 10 to 20 month-old infants were not getting enough vitamin D from supplements, or possibly not enough sunshine (*ibid,* 51 [1990]: 202-208).

Regarding iron, eating foods rich in vitamin C at each meal will help enhance the absorption of iron from the diet. The vegetarian usually does eat plenty of fruit or vegetables with each meal, so this is generally not a problem.

What about protein? The American Dietetic Association has concluded that "mixtures of proteins from grains, vegetables, legumes, seeds, and nuts eaten over the course of the day complement one another in their amino acid profiles without the necessity of precise planning and complementation of proteins within each meal, as the recently popular combined proteins theory" has urged. In other words, protein is readily available in plant foods, and there is absolutely no need to worry about getting enough of it.

During rapid growth, lactation, or recovery from illness, the lacto-ovovegetarian diet can meet all the nutrient requirements if enough total food is eaten. For the vegan, care must be taken during these stressful times to take in enough calories, vitamin B_{12}, and vitamin D.

In general, the lacto-ovovegetarian diet is not only safe, but helps an individual conform more closely to healthful guidelines for eating. The vegan diet can also be safe and very healthful if a wide variety of foods are consumed and vitamin B_{12} supplements used.

Economic and Ecological

"Vegetarianism has three things going for it all at once— economics, health, and compassion" (Dr. Jean Mayer).

The argument here is that raising animals for food requires high amounts of land, water, and plant feed, and with world hunger we need to maximize our resources so that more can be fed.

At present there are 5 billion people in the world, with about 4 billion living in developing Third World countries. Economists say that food production in less developed countries will barely keep pace with population growth, which will reduce the reserves needed to combat malnutrition, hunger, and disease.

In developed countries, where the food supply is overabundant, the main problem is overnutrition, which leads to obesity, heart disease, cancer, and diabetes.

As Dr. Robert Olson of the State University of New York at Buffalo has recently concluded, "All countries could cooperate to overcome hunger and malnutrition, prevent diseases of overnutrition, and improve the overall quality of life on this planet" (*Nutrition Today*, January/February 1989).

For example, if one were to grow corn and feed it directly to humans, more people could be fed than if the corn were fed to a cow, and then its milk or flesh consumed. For every 3,000 calories of corn fed to a cow, only 600 are returned in milk, and if the meat is consumed, only 120 calories are available for human consumption. For every 10 pounds of corn protein fed to a cow, only one pound is returned in the form of meat. When soybeans are grown on an acre of land, 450 pounds of protein are produced. This is in contrast to only 40 pounds of pork or 45 pounds of beef for the same acre of land.

Obviously, more people can be fed when humans use plant food as opposed to animal products. Other economic issues are also at stake. For example, meats are six times as expensive as flour, cereal, potatoes, and legumes when considering overall nutritional value.

In one study, conducted in 1990, a diet low in saturated fat and cholesterol (low amounts of meat or fatty dairy products) was calculated to save the consumer $230 each year (*Circulation* 81 [1990]: 1721-1733). Also, because saturated fats and cholesterol (which are high in meat and dairy products) have been associated with heart disease, cancer, and other diseases, we all end up paying indirectly through increased health insurance premiums and taxes.

Ethical

"I hold flesh food to be unsuited to our species. We err in copying the lower animal world if we are superior to it" (Mahatma Gandhi).

Many vegetarians claim this as their number one motivation.

Taking the lives of animals and then eating their flesh appears cruel to some people.

During the early 1800s in the United States, ethical motives for being a vegetarian were promoted strongly. As Dr. James Whorton has written: "Before the 1830s the concern of vegetarians was to save animals, and afterward it was to save people. . . . From the ancients (Pythagoras and Porphyry in particular) came the idea that the killing and eating of beasts contaminated and brutalized the human soul. . . . Savagery could be manifested not only by inhumanity to man, but by cruelty toward animals as well'' (*Crusaders for Fitness*, p. 65).

In the words of Ellen White: ''What man with a human heart, who has ever cared for domestic animals, could look into their eyes, so full of confidence and affection, and willingly give them over to the butcher's knife?'' (*The Ministry of Healing*, pp. 316, 317).

Many Americans are repulsed at the suffering some animals go through in the name of research. Some are just as upset with the way animals are crowded close together in uncomfortable pens prior to death, and then slain so that their flesh may be eaten.

Fitness

''In 1896 the aptly named James Parsley led the Vegetarian Cycling Club to easy victory over two regular clubs. A week later he won the most prestigious hill-climbing race in England, breaking the hill record by nearly a minute. Other members of the club also turned in remarkable performances. Their competitors were having to eat crow with their beef'' (James C. Whorton).

The relationship between vegetarian dietary practices and performance has a long and colorful history. The ancient Greek athletes were heavy meat eaters. Milo of Croton, the legendary Greek wrestler who was never once brought to his knees over five Olympiads (532-516 B.C.), supposedly consumed gargantuan amounts of meat. The Greek concept of the importance of meat for performance still lingers.

During the mid-1800s Dr. Justus von Liebig, the preeminent physiological chemist of his time, promoted the concept that energy for all muscular movement came from protein. Most heavy laborers and athletes were found to be eating diets high in protein, and this was accepted by nutritionists at that time as a physical necessity. Since the typical meatless diet was thought to contain insufficient quantities of protein, vegetarians were thought to be theoretically incapable of prolonged exercise.

Undaunted, vegetarians of the 1800s sought to prove,

through excellence in endurance exercise, the superiority of the plant-based diet. During the 1890s the London Vegetarian Society formed an athletic and cycling club. As noted in the beginning quote, James Parsley and the other 90 members of the club vindicated their diet, outperforming their carnivorous competitors.

American vegetarian cyclists also demonstrated their abilities. Will Brown, who in the 1890s switched to a vegetarian diet for health reasons, went on to thrash all records for the 2,000-mile bicycle race. Margarita Gast established a women's record for 1,000 miles on a vegetarian diet.

Other vegetarian athletes joined in the foray. Long distance walking races were also very popular in the 1890s, and were regarded then as the ultimate test of endurance. In the 1893 race from Berlin to Vienna, the first two competitors to cover the 372-mile course were vegetarians. A 100-kilometer race held several years later in Germany also attracted much attention, with 11 of the first 14 finishers being vegetarian.

Many other vegetarian athletes performed amazingly well. In 1912 the vegetarian Kolehmainen became one of the first men to complete the marathon under 2:30. Other records were set by vegetarian swimmers, tennis players, and other athletes, including the West Ham Vegetarian Society's undefeated tug-of-war team.

A few simple early studies attempted to measure the ability of vegetarian athletes. The Belgian researcher Dr. Schouteden carried out tests in 1904 on 25 students divided into vegetarian and meat-eating groups. For each he determined the endurance of the forearm muscles by measuring the maximum number of times each subject could lift a weight on a pulley by squeezing a handle. The mean number of contractions for vegetarians was 69, for meat eaters 38.

Irving Fisher of Yale University in 1906 reported on his study of Yale athletes trained on a full flesh diet, athletes who abstained from meat, and sedentary vegetarians (nurses and physicians from the Battle Creek Sanitarium). Each was tested to determine the maximum length of time that the arms could be held out horizontally. The maximum number of deep knee bends and leg raises was also measured. The final tally for all tests was heavily in favor of the vegetarians. In the horizontal arm hold test, only two of the 15 meat eaters were able to maintain the arm hold more than 15 minutes, and none achieved a half hour. Of the vegetarians, however, 22 of 32 exceeded 15 minutes, 15 broke the 30 minute barrier, 9 broke 60 minutes, and one surpassed 3 hours.

Other researchers have focused their efforts on the functional capacities of primitive peoples consuming vegetarian diets. The Tarahumara Indians, a Ute-Aztecan tribe living in the rugged Sierra Madre Occidental Mountains in the north central state of Chihuahua, Mexico, have been studied extensively. They are known for their extraordinary physical fitness and endurance as long-distance runners. Unusual stamina has characterized the Tarahumara Indians from the earliest recorded descriptions. It is best demonstrated in their popular sport called raripuri, in which participants race 150-300 kilometers kicking a wooden ball.

Their simple, near-vegetarian diet, composed primarily of corn and beans (90 percent of total calories), provides them with 75-80 percent of total calories in the form of carbohydrate, and appears to be one factor explaining their exceptional ability to engage in endurance exercise.

Today we know that the superior performance of some of the early vegetarian athletes is probably best explained not only by their motivation to demonstrate excellence, but also by their higher carbohydrate intakes. Carbohydrate is present in large quantities in grains, potatoes, dried fruit, and other plant foods, but is virtually nonexistent in meat. Research from both Europe and the United States has supported the concept that carbohydrate promotes endurance performance in such activities as running, swimming, and cycling.

Athletes who use high amounts of carbohydrates have greater levels of muscle glycogen. This allows them to exercise up to three times longer before exhaustion. For this reason, most endurance athletes today "carbohydrate-load" during hard training and before competitive events.

Concluding Remarks

For all the reasons reviewed in this chapter—spiritual, health and disease prevention, nutritional, economical and ecological, ethical, and fitness—the vegetarian diet stands head and shoulders above all other types of eating patterns. The vegetarian diet truly is the diet for all time, both on this earth and the new one to come.

CHAPTER 7

Health
and the Mind

"I thank and praise you, O God of my fathers,
for you have given me wisdom
and glowing health."—Daniel 2:23, TLB.

Plain Living, High Thinking?

During the first captivity in 605 B.C., as Judah was slowly falling apart under the sieges of Babylon, Daniel, age 18, and other young princes of royal blood were chosen to be trained for government service under Nebuchadnezzar. Being members of the royal school, the youth were given food and drink from the royal household. Most pious Jews would probably want to avoid such food because the meats were, in some instances, from unclean animals that had first been offered to pagan gods. Additionally, Daniel's 10-day food request implies that he desired a plain and healthful vegetarian diet.

Daniel, whose name means "God is my judge," "resolved not to defile himself with the royal food and wine, and he asked the chief official for permission not to defile himself this way" (Daniel 1:8, NIV). When the official expressed concern that Daniel and his friends might end up "looking worse than the other young men" (verse 10, NIV) if they avoided the royal food, Daniel proposed a 10-day research project.

"Please test your servants for ten days: Give us nothing but vegetables to eat and water to drink. Then compare our appearance with that of the young men who eat the royal food, and treat your servants in accordance with what you see" (verses 12, 13, NIV).

Daniel and his companions passed the test with flying colors. "At the end of the ten days they looked healthier and better nourished than any of the young men who ate the royal food. So the guard took away their choice food and the wine they were to drink and gave them vegetables instead" (verses 15, 16, NIV).

In the very next verse we are told that God gave these men "knowledge and understanding of all kinds of literature and learning" (verse 17, NIV).

Plain living and high thinking—is there a connection? Daniel's experience would most certainly lead us to make such a conclusion. Let's review what science has discovered on this issue.

Diet, Brain, and Behavior

"What you eat today will be walking and talking tomorrow" (Jack LaLanne).

The developed human brain is composed of approximately 100 billion nerve cells (neurons) and even more supporting cells (glia). Even though the brain comprises only 2 percent of adult body weight, it receives 15 percent of the blood pumped out of the heart and accounts for 20 to 30 percent of the oxygen used by the body at rest. The constant electrical activity of the brain probably accounts for most of the brain's energy requirements. Unlike other organs of the body, the brain does not store carbohydrate or fat for energy. Thus, it is heavily dependent upon a constant supply of oxygen and glucose from the blood. As a result, it is not surprising that brain function is relatively sensitive to the quality of the diet.

Brain cells, or neurons, use many chemicals to communicate with each other and to send messages to the rest of the body. Between 30 and 40 of these chemicals, known as neurotransmitters, have been identified. These chemicals help brain messages to jump the small space (called the synapse) between brain cells.

Amazingly enough, the creation of these neurotransmitters depends on enzyme systems that use vitamins and minerals from the diet. Also, many amino acids from the protein of the diet are used by the brain to make the neurotransmitters. In other words, nutrients from the diet can affect the formation of the chemical messengers of your brain!

Although research in this area is still very limited, food is known to affect the way the brain functions. Here is one of the best researched examples. One of the brain chemical messengers is called serotonin. The brain cells use one of the essential amino acids called tryptophan to make serotonin. When you eat high amounts of sugar (carbohydrate), the brain has an easier time in drawing tryptophan from the blood into the brain. More than the normal amount of serotonin is formed by the brain cells, and this makes humans feel sleepy. On the other hand, high protein, low carbohydrate meals tend to increase the amount of the amino acid tyrosine going into the brain, promoting brain formation of the neurotransmitter catecholamine. This may make some people feel more alert (*Nutrition Review* 44 [1986]: 2-6).

Many nutrients, including vitamin B_6, iron, vitamin C, copper, and zinc, are known to aid the brain cells in making neurotransmitters. Some researchers have shown that when iron is low in the diet, some people change their normal behavior. In children, for example, low amounts of iron have been associated with apathy, short attention span, irritability, and reduced ability to learn. For example, children who are iron-deficient become less alert. In addition, if infants survive starvation, or what is called protein-calorie malnutrition, lasting impairments in behavior and cognition can result.

New evidence shows that the type of fat you eat in your diet influences the quality of the membrane around brain cells. This may affect the activity of the enzymes of the brain cell, which may then affect neurotransmitter formation. Research in the future will help us understand what type of dietary fat is best.

Diet and Abnormal Behavior

Because of these preliminary findings, there has been much discussion concerning the link between diet and abnormal behavior in both children and adults. Could it be true that individuals who behave abnormally are eating poorly?

Advocates claim that criminals commit crimes because of deficient diets. In response to these theories, correctional facilities in several states have actually gone so far as to change the diets of inmates, provide megavitamin supplements, and begin testing for low blood glucose levels and food allergies.

The belief that diet has a major influence on criminal behavior has already made its way into the courtroom. The most famous example of this was the "Twinkie defense" in the Dan White murder trial. Dan White was a former San Francisco supervisor who went to the city hall with a loaded gun, climbed through a window to avoid a metal detector, and then killed both Mayor George Moscone and Supervisor Harvey Milk.

On the surface, it appeared to be a clear case of premeditated murder, but White's attorney used a "diminished capacity" defense to argue that White's ability to "maturely and meaningfully" reflect on the evil nature of his intended action was impaired as a result of depression. White's "penchant for wolfing down junk food—Twinkies, Cokes, doughnuts, and candy bars . . . exacerbated his depression and indicated a chemical imbalance of the brain" (*ibid.*, pp. 89-94). As a result, White was given a reduced sentence of manslaughter, creating tremendous public controversy.

The belief that sugar causes behavior and learning problems in children is widely held by the general public. Popular interest in this position has been heightened by media reports of the "Halloween effect" and the writings of the late Dr. Ben Feingold. In 1973 Dr. Feingold, a California allergist, proposed that artifical flavors and food colors were a cause of hyperactivity in children (*Pediatrics* 66 [1980]: 521-525). Dr. Feingold recommended a diet free of these substances as both treatment and prevention of the condition. He published two popular books on the subject, *Why Your Child Is Hyperactive* (1974) and *The Feingold Cookbook for Hyperactive Children* (1979).

Others later urged that sugar also was a factor explaining hyperactivity and aggression in children. Many parents adopted the diet for their "hyperactive" children, and beliefs persist to this day that Feingold's writings are accurate.

However, well-controlled, double-blind studies have not been able to show that children thought to be hyperactive are actually affected when sugar, artificial food dyes, or other food additives are added to meals. In one study, children who were believed by their parents to have adverse responses to sugar were brought to a clinic for seven sessions. During each session, varying levels of either aspartame (Nutrasweet) or sugar in water were fed to the children. However, neither the researchers nor the children knew which sweetener they were consuming. A complex series of physical and psychological tests showed no effect of sugar on behavior. Other similar tests with food dyes and food additives have also shown no negative effects on behavior (*Nutrition Review* 44 [1986]: 144-150).

Studies on changes in the diets of inmates are also unsupportive. It appears that the diet has to be abnormally extreme to produce any meaningful change in behavior. Although there is plenty of evidence showing that substances from the diet can have subtle effects on human behavior, and that brain chemicals are derived from the diet, there is no support for the theory that abnormal behavior (criminal, hyperactivity) can be traced to the diet.

Conclusion

The information in this chapter suggests that diet has subtle but measurable effects on the brain, influencing how a person feels. Until research leads us further, most reviewers on this topic suggest that a well-balanced, healthy diet be consumed to ensure that the brain receives an optimal supply of nutrients.

However, we should not go to the other extreme and assume that mischievous and criminal behavior by children and adults is entirely explained by junk-food diets. Many other factors are involved, including the influence of family, friends, neighbors, and colleagues; other factors in the lifestyle, including insufficient exercise or excessive mental stress; or one's relationship with God.

CHAPTER 8

Lessons From the Olympic Games

"Do you not know that in a race all the
runners run, but only one gets the prize?
Run in such a way as to get the prize." —
1 Corinthians 9:24, NIV.

The apostle Paul appears to have been quite knowledgeable about the Olympic Games of his time and era. As we will see later in this chapter, he was fond of using imagery from the games to help his readers better understand various spiritual truths. Let's first review what the ancient Greek Olympic Games were like.

Milo

Milo of Croton, the greatest of the ancient Greek athletes, earned his legendary fame as a mighty, fearless wrestler. With three falls to the knees constituting defeat, Milo was never once brought to his knees in five Olympiads, nine Nemean, ten Isthmian, and six Pythian games.

Milo started his intensive training four years before his first Olympics in 532 B.C. Each day, so the story goes, Milo would lift his baby bull to his shoulders and walk as far as he could. This continued week after week, month after month, with Milo increasing in strength and size as his bull increased in weight.

After four years of this regimen, Milo went to his first Olympics, bringing his bull along. To impress the gathered athletes and spectators, Milo sacrificed his faithful bull, and then carried the massive carcass 400 meters around the stadium on his shoulders.

Later Milo wrestled to victory, starting his illustrious athletic career. He soon became a Greek hero, and was adored by the populace, with statues erected in his honor, and odes written for his glorification.

Greek Physical Culture and the Olympic Games

The story of Milo typifies the ancient Greek love of athletics. From the end of the Homeric age (750 B.C.) throughout the era of Greek city-states (fifth century B.C.) to the rapid and wide conquests of Alexander the Great (323 B.C.) to the final subjugation to Roman power (31 B.C.) and beyond to the reign of the Christian emperor Theodosius I (A.D. 393), athletics and physical training remained a steadfast core of Greek culture.

The ancient Greek Olympic Games began in 776 B.C., approximately 30 years before Isaiah began his reign as Israel's prophet. The Games were held every four years and continued without interruption for more than 1,000 years, despite the negative influence of the conquering Romans. The Olympic Games finally ended in A.D. 393 when the Christian emperor Theodosius I ordered that all pagan cults and centers be closed.

Religious ceremonies occupied a substantial part of the five-day period of the games, one of the major reasons these games and others were found intolerable by Christians.

The first day of the ancient Olympics was devoted to the worship of Zeus and other Greek gods. The morning of the third day was reserved for more religious ceremony, culminating in the sacrifice of 100 oxen on the great altar of Zeus, the chief Greek god. When the program was completed on the fifth and final day, there were other sacrifices and thank offerings.

The competitors swore by Zeus that they would obey the rules and play fair. They prayed to Zeus for "either the wreath or death." To the Greeks, there was no separation of church and state, no line between the sacred and the secular. There was no inconsistency between worship and fiercely competitive games as parts of a religious festival.

The Greeks had a polytheistic religion—the various gods were viewed as immortal and superhuman, but at the same time quite human in that they ate, drank, and quarreled among themselves.

The Greek gods were seen as patrons of success, not creators. Success was assisted by divine favor, but application, hard work, and self-reliance were seen as keys to victory. So the gods were placated and honored with sacrifices, libations, and festivals, but not depended upon.

Victory alone brought glory. Participation entailed no virtue. Defeat brought undying shame. In the ancient Games, there were no second or third awards, as there are today. Not to be first was to lose. This is why the competitors prayed for either the wreath or death. The slogan of the Greek athletes was ''always to be first and to surpass the others.''

Every four years the athletes came to Olympia, a hilly, agrarian site in the Greek district of Elis. They arrived one month early to train under strict supervision, after swearing to Zeus that they had already been training all of 10 months.

After the first day of religious services, the second day opened with the chariot race and horse race. The same day the pentathlon was conducted in the stadium where naked men, according to strict and specific rules, threw the discus and javelin, wrestled, ran the 200-meter sprint, and participated in the standing long jump.

Three running events were held during the morning of the fourth day—the 200-, 400-, and 4,800-meter events. Three exceedingly brutal, violent, and popular events were reserved for the afternoon—wrestling, boxing, and the pankration (a mixture of boxing, wrestling, and kicking).

In wrestling, three falls to the knees constituted defeat. Biting and gouging were prohibited, but not much else. Boxers wore leather thongs wound tightly round the hands and wrists. They fought, with no breaks, until one was knocked out or raised his hand. There was terrible bloodiness, with death one of the recognized risks.

The number one Olympian sport was the pankration. One "surrendered" by tapping the victor on the back or shoulder. Contestants punched, slapped, and purposely broke the opponent's toe and finger bones.

All Olympic winners received the coveted Olympic wreath, fashioned from the branches of a sacred olive tree. The winners were well rewarded by their native cities, honored in celebrations, banquets, and triumphal processions. Often a breach was made in the wall of the hometown. Sculptors carved the winner's figure in stone, poets wrote odes commemorating his achievements.

While the populace by and large enjoyed the Games, a narrow circle of intellectuals, moralists, and philosophers were vocal in their criticism, with a battle of words waging between them and the athletes. Criticism was based on two views. One was that the glorification of the athlete rested on the false evaluation of what is truly and properly human, exaggerating bodily excellences at the expense of mental and spiritual progress. The other view was that enthusiasm for the victors and the Games diverted attention and energy from the real needs of the community.

For these reasons, Aristotle cautioned:

"The athlete's habit of body neither produces a good condition for the general purposes of civic life, nor does it encourage ordinary health and the procreation of children. . . . Some amount of exertion is essential for the best habit, but it must be neither violent nor specialized, as is the case with the athlete. It should rather be a general exertion, directed to all the activities of a free man."

Other philosophers liked to poke fun at the athletes. Diogenes the Cynic once met an athlete celebrating with his friends, boasting that he was the fastest runner in all of Greece. Diogenes dismissed him in one sentence, "But not faster than a rabbit or a deer, and they, the swiftest of the animals, are also the most cowardly."

There were some philosophers, however, who defended the athletes. Pindar, the great Boeotian lyric poet, felt that the virtues of discipline and endurance as displayed by the athletes were ennobling, reflecting greatness of soul.

Paul's True Olympians

The apostle Paul, while not condoning the Greek Games, did use them as a tool to better portray various Christian concepts. Paul, as was Pindar, was enamored by the single-hearted purpose, perseverance, and endurance displayed by the athletes, referring to this many times. (See 1 Corinthians 9:24-27; Hebrews 12:1-12; Philippians 3:13, 14; 2 Timothy 2:5; Galatians 5:7.)

Paul, however, strongly reasoned that the goal should be something far greater than the fame associated with the olive wreath crown "that will not last" (1 Corinthians 9:25, NIV). The goal, wrote Paul, is a "crown that will last forever," (verse 25, NIV), which is "the life to come" (1 Timothy 4:8, NIV), "the eternal life to which you were called" (1 Timothy 6:12, NIV), "the prize for which God has called me heavenward in Christ Jesus" (Philippians 3:14, NIV).

In aiming for this goal, however, cautioned Paul, the process does not involve being competitive against others, but striving with others as we "fix our eyes on Jesus" (Hebrews 12:2, NIV). We are to do nothing "out of selfish ambition or vain conceit, but in humility consider others better" than ourselves (Philippians 2:3, NIV). Instead of comparing ourselves with others (Galatians 6:4), we are to contend "as one man for the faith of the gospel," (Philippians 1:27, NIV), honoring one another above ourselves (Romans 12:10).

Very important, God is not seen as the patron of our success and strength, but the source. Paul wrote, in God "we live and move and have our being" (Acts 17:28). Success depends not on man's "desire or effort, but on God's mercy" (Romans 9:16, NIV), for we can only do "everything through him who gives" us strength (Philippians 4:13, NIV).

So in contrast to the Greeks, Paul pointed out that true Olympians have a single-hearted desire for something greater, that is eternal life and godliness. In striving for this goal, we depend totally on God as the source of energy and strength, giving Him the praise for success, as we work with others and for others, not against them.

Aesop, a philosopher on the island of Samos during the sixth century B.C., once met a boastful victor in one of the body-contact sports. Aesop asked him whether the opponent he had defeated was the stronger man of the two. "Don't say that," replied the athlete. "My strength proved to be much greater." "Well then, you simpleton," said Aesop, "what honor have you earned if, being the stronger, you prevailed over a weaker man? You might be tolerated if you were telling us that by skill you overcame a man who was superior to you in bodily strength."

Aesop points out in this dialogue the irrational basis of human competition. The apostle Paul lifts us above such behavior, leading us to depend on the everlasting arms of strength, thus empowering us to lift others higher—the true spirit of real Olympians.

CHAPTER 9

The Benefits
of Smoking Cessation

---

*"A custom loathsome to the eye, harmful to the
brain, dangerous to the lungs, and in the black,
stinking fume thereof, nearest resembling the
horrible Stygian smoke of the pit that is bottomless."—
James I of England, 1604.*

On the overall issue of appetite, Seventh-day Adventists have traditionally made a division between substances that should never be used (tobacco, alcohol, and drugs), those that should be consumed moderately, with care against excess (dietary fats, sugar, eggs, salt), and those that should be freely ingested on a daily basis for health (fruits, vegetables, and whole grains).

The Bible is replete with advice on the importance of moderation and self-control, typified by the text "Blessed are you, O land whose king is of noble birth and whose princes eat at a proper time—for strength and not for drunkenness" (Ecclesiastes 10:17, NIV).

The apostle Paul lays down a central guiding principle on the entire issue of health and appetite: "Do you not know that your body is a temple of the Holy Spirit, who is in you, whom you have received from God? You are not your own; you were bought at a price. Therefore honor God with your body" (1 Corinthians 6:19, 20, NIV).

In no area of health is this principle more important and applicable than that of cigarette smoking. Smoking is the most deleterious public health problem of our era. Seventh-day Adventists have for decades been at the forefront of community smoking cessation efforts, and this chapter will give additional information to those who continue in the fight for a smoke-free society.

The Early History of Tobacco

The fight against tobacco began when it was first introduced in Europe in the fifteenth century. Rodrigo de Jerez, a member of Christopher Columbus' expedition, who apparently learned to smoke in Cuba, lit up for the first time back home in Spain. The townspeople—alarmed by the smoke issuing from his mouth and nose—assumed he had been possessed by the devil. He was promptly imprisoned, and thus began the battle to eradicate smoking from civilized society.

King James I of England considered tobacco and papism to be among the biggest evils facing his realm (see the quote at the beginning of this chapter). Several popes agreed with him, at least on the first point. Pope Innocent X and Pope Urban VIII excommunicated smokers. In China smokers were decapitated; in Russia they were flogged.

The first organized antitobacco movement in the United States began in the 1830s, led by health reformer Sylvester Graham. But it was largely a losing battle, as many physicians actually recommended smoking for health back then.

Belief in the healing power of tobacco dates back to the sixteenth century. The idea was promoted that Native Americans enjoyed better health than Europeans because they were protected by their smoking habit.

By the 1880s, however, antismoking forces had regrouped, in response to the threat posed by a new enemy—the cigarette manufacturing machine. Although crude cigarettes had been available long before, the development, in 1881, of a workable cigarette manufacturing machine brought an increase in sales as the retail price dropped. Suddenly cigarettes were available to the masses.

Antismoking forces made claims that cigarettes were spiked

with opium, wrapped in paper that had been whitened with arsenic, unhealthy and even fatal, and were corrupting American youth. Efforts to curb smoking by minors served as the opening wedge in the legislative campaign against cigarettes.

By 1890, according to one tally, 26 states and territories had outlawed the sale of cigarettes to minors (age 14 to 24 years). Around the turn of the century, 14 states had even outlawed the sale of cigarettes to adults.

Congress was asked to protect the public health by requiring that cigarette packages be stamped with a skull and crossbones and labeled "poison." Many employers refused to hire cigarette smokers. Nonsmokers said their health was being jeopardized by "secondhand smoke."

World War I provided the nails for the coffin of the first anticigarette movement. Increased prosperity, the demands of the military, and the spread of cigarette smoking among women combined to strengthen the industry while weakening the opposition.

Military commanders had long regarded tobacco as essential for the fighting man, and a national campaign was organized to ensure that each man in the military had free cigarettes. By the time Johnny came marching home, the cigarette had become an almost unassailable symbol of courage, decency, and the American way.

Toward a Tobacco-free Society

"The public health impact of smoking is enormous. An estimated 390,000 Americans die each year from disease caused by smoking. More than one of every six deaths in the United States is caused by smoking" (Dr. Antonia Novello, surgeon general of the United States).

Although the cigarette won the first round, out of the ashes of the old antismoking movement has come a new campaign that has been so successful that it may lead in the near future to a society that is largely smoke-free. Smoking used to be chic—now it's shunned. The ashtray is following the spittoon into oblivion.

One of the biggest leaders in the smoke-free society movement has been Dr. C. Everett Koop, former surgeon general of the United States. In 1989 he wrote, "Because the general health risks of smoking are well known, because smoking is banned or restricted in a growing number of public places and worksites, and because smoking is losing its social acceptability, the overall prevalence of smoking in our society is likely to continue to decline. The progress we have achieved during the past quarter century is impressive."

During the early 1960s, the Advisory Committee on Smoking and Health to the Surgeon General was formed to study the health consequences of smoking. After more than one year of study the final report of the advisory committee was released on January 11, 1964. It concluded that "cigarette smoking is causally related to lung cancer in men; the magnitude of the effect of cigarette smoking far outweighs all other factors."

This was an about-face from a report published 16 years before in the *Journal of the American Medical Association* that argued "more can be said in behalf of smoking as a form of escape from tension than against it. . . . There does not seem to be any preponderance of evidence that would indicate the abolition of the use of tobacco as a substance contrary to the public health."

Knowledge of the health consequences of smoking has expanded dramatically since 1964, and 10 key findings and occurrences during the past quarter century include the following:

1. Smoking is responsible for more than one of every six deaths in the United States and remains the single most important preventable cause of death in our society.

2. More than 390,000 deaths each year are related to cigarette smoking, led by heart disease (115,000 deaths/year), lung cancer (106,000), other lung diseases (57,000), and stroke (27,500). To date, 43 chemicals in tobacco smoke have been determined to cause cancer. Smoking during pregnancy accounts for 10 percent of all infant deaths. Many smoking-related deaths occur before age 65, striking people in the prime of their life.

3. The prevalence of smoking among adults decreased from 40 percent in 1965 to 26 percent in 1991. The U.S. Public Health Service's goal is that only 15 percent of Americans will be smoking in the year 2000. Nearly half of all living adults who ever smoked have quit, representing more than 38 million. However, 50 million Americans continue to smoke.

4. Since 1964 more than 750,000 smoking-related deaths were avoided or postponed as a result of decisions by people to quit smoking or not to start.

5. The prevalence of smoking remains higher among Blacks, blue-collar workers, and less-educated people than in the overall population. The decline in smoking has been substantially slower among women than among men.

6. Smoking begins primarily during childhood and adolescence. The age of initiation has fallen over time, especially among females. One quarter of high school seniors who have ever smoked had their first cigarette by sixth grade, one-half by eighth grade. More than 3,000 teenagers become regular smokers each day. There is a growing consensus that smoking prevention education needs to begin in elementary school.

7. Considerable evidence exists that many adverse health effects are related to passive smoking (breathing someone else's cigarette smoke). These include an increased risk for cancer, heart disease, and other lung disorders. The children of parents who smoke compared with the children of nonsmoking parents have an increased frequency of lung infections and symptoms.

Several studies have shown that the simple separation of smokers and nonsmokers within the same air space may reduce, but does not eliminate, the exposure of nonsmokers to environmental tobacco smoke.

8. As of mid-1988, more than 320 local communities had adopted laws or regulations restricting smoking in public places, a threefold increase in three years. Much of this is owing to public outcry against the health dangers of passive smoking.

9. There is increasing evidence that the use of economic incentives, such as excise taxation of tobacco products, work-

place financial benefits, and insurance premium differentials for smokers and nonsmokers, discourages use of tobacco.

10. Among the key challenges for the future are these obstacles: the highly addictive nature of tobacco (nicotine is six to eight times more addictive than alcohol); the high rate of relapse for those who try to quit (less than 10 percent of those who try to quit do it successfully); the fact that cigarettes are among the most heavily advertised products in society; the prominent role of tobacco in the agricultural economy of several states (for example, in North Carolina, where 56 percent of all U.S. cigarettes are made, tobacco provides $7.3 billion for the state economy and one out of every 11 jobs).

The Benefits of Quitting

"Quitting smoking carries major and immediate health benefits for men and women of all ages, even those in the older age groups" (Dr. Antonia Novello).

In 1990 Dr. Antonia Novello released a landmark document entitled *The Health Benefits of Smoking Cessation*. This was the first surgeon general's report to provide a comprehensive statement on this topic. The value of the information in this report is that people often respond better to evidence that outlines the benefits of changing their behavior than descriptions of the negative and dire consequences (scare tactics).

It is urged that the information from this report be used in all smoking cessation programs by the church. Several key items from this report include:

● After an ex-smoker stays off cigarettes for 15 years, the risk of death returns to nearly the level of people who never smoked. The risk of heart disease falls by 50 percent after just one year, while risk of lung cancer falls 30-50 percent after 10 years of abstinence.

● Male and female smokers who quit between ages 35 and 39

add an average of five and three years to their lives, respectively. Quitting at ages 65 to 69 adds one full year of life.

● Ex-smokers compared to smokers have fewer days of illness, fewer health complaints, better overall health status, and fewer lung problems.

● Nicotine withdrawal symptoms peak in the first one to two days after quitting and subside rapidly during the following weeks. Symptoms include anxiety, irritability, frustration, anger, difficulty concentrating, and restlessness.

● The average weight gain after quitting smoking is only five pounds. Very few gain excessive amounts of weight. The health benefits of quitting far exceed any risks from the average five-pound weight gain. Weight gain can be limited by satisfying cravings with small pieces of fruit or vegetables instead of sugary and fatty foods and snacks, drinking six to eight glasses of water per day, and walking 30 minutes a day.

● Most ex-smokers try to quit more than once before they succeed. Two thirds of smokers say they would like to quit, and only 19 percent have never tried to quit. Each year more than 1 million smokers quit successfully, 90 percent of them on their own as a result of social pressures, personal reasons, etc. However, only 10 percent of those who try to quit are successful. With good smoking cessation programs (such as Breathe Free), 20 percent to 40 percent are able to quit smoking and stay off cigarettes for at least one year.

Concluding Remarks

Charles Lamb in *A Farewell to Tobacco*, quipped, "For thy sake, tobacco, I would do anything but die." As pointed out in this chapter, however, the tobacco user ends up having little choice in the matter. We are "fearfully and wonderfully made"

(Psalm 139:14), and the decision not to smoke cigarettes most certainly allows us to better ''honor God'' in our bodies (1 Corinthians 6:20, NIV).

CHAPTER 10

Stress
Management

"No wind favors him who has no destined port." —
Montaigne.

Jacob was born second to Esau, holding his hairy brother's heel, and was thus named Jacob, "the deceiver" (Genesis 25:26). When he was 15, his beloved grandfather Abraham died, from whom Jacob learned that the birthright should pass on to Esau. This began a long period of stressful years as Jacob deceived, retreated, and struggled with Esau over this issue.

During his 20-year exile Jacob stayed with Laban, the selfish, crooked brother of his mother, and fell in love with Rachel, for whom he worked seven long, hard years. Because of the duplicity of Laban, Jacob ended up having to marry Leah, the sister of Rachel, and working another seven years for the woman he really wanted.

While working for Laban, Jacob had 11 sons and one daughter by his two wives and their two maidservants, creating a family admixture that resulted in untold grief for Jacob and the entire household (Genesis 30).

The rivalry between the two sisters was intense, and each of the 11 sons received a name reflecting the contention between them. The early negative influence of Laban, 33 years of life in heathen Canaan, the favoritism of Jacob for the sons of Rachel, and the loss of Joseph created a home with envy, jealousy, discord, and misery. This atmosphere often predominated any semblance of religious zeal and lofty faith.

During his years of exile, Jacob also suffered deep mental anguish because of the shame of his sin of deceiving his father. Not until the night when he wrestled with God by the brook Jabbok did he experience the spiritual rebirth symbolized by his name change to Israel (Genesis 32:28).

Quite a stressful life! When Jacob was brought by Joseph to meet Pharaoh 17 years before his death, "Pharaoh asked him, 'How old are you?' And Jacob said to Pharaoh, 'The years of my pilgrimage are a hundred and thirty. My years have been few and difficult, and they do not equal the years of the pilgrimage of my fathers' " (Genesis 47:8, 9, NIV).

The Meaning of Stress

Stress has been defined as any action or situation (stressors) that places special physical or psychological demands upon an individual—in other words, anything that unbalances one's equilibrium.

Dr. Hans Selye, one of the great pioneers of medicine and the originator of the concept of stress, in his famous 1956 classic, *The Stress of Life*, wrote, "In its medical sense, stress is essentially the rate of wear and tear in the body . . . the nonspecific response of the body to any demand."

In Dr. Selye's view, both good and bad stressors produce stress reactions in the body. A divorce is stressful—but so is getting married. Both upset an individual's equilibrium and require adjustment and adaptation.

But it is not the stressor itself that creates the response. It is the person's reaction to the stressor. Therefore individuals will have varying responses to the same stressor, based on their own characteristic response.

Medical research on stress dates back to the 1920s, when Walter Cannon began experimenting with the physiological effect of stress on cats and dogs. Studying the animals' reactions to danger, the Harvard physiologist noted a regular and common pattern, now known as the fight-or-flight response.

In this response, the muscles tense and tighten, breathing becomes deeper and faster, the heart rate rises and blood vessels constrict, raising the blood pressure, the stomach and intestines temporarily halt digestion, perspiration increases, while the secretion of saliva and mucus decrease, the sense organs sharpen perception, and the thyroid is stimulated. Various stress hormones, in particular epinephrine and cortisol, increase in the body, depressing immune function and causing many other negative effects.

In the 1940s and 1950s, Dr. Selye, working as a researcher at Montreal's Institute of Experimental Medicine and Surgery, extended Cannon's work and laid the foundation for much of today's research on stress. Experimenting with rats, he used various stressors, and found that a regular pattern of responses occurred, described as the general adaptation syndrome (alarm, resistance, exhaustion).

He discovered that if the stressor was maintained for a prolonged period of time, the body would first go through an alarm reaction (fight-or-flight responses outlined above), followed by a stage of resistance in which body functions would return close to normal as the body strove to resist the stress. Finally, there would be a stage of exhaustion, in which the symptoms of the alarm reaction returned. In animal experiments, the animals would die.

In chapter 11 we will review some of the many studies that have shown that illness and early death from heart disease and cancer occur in people who are chronically anxious, depressed, or who suffer other stress-related problems over a long period of time.

Even on a short-term basis, high levels of stress have been associated with increased risk of getting flus and colds. The immune system cannot function as well when the mind is feeling stressed. For example, separated and divorced women have been found to have much higher rates of infectious diseases than married women. More on all this in chapter 11. In this chapter, we'll consider techniques for stress management.

According to a series of national surveys conducted by Louis Harris and Associates for *Prevention* magazine, between the years of 1983 and 1990, the percentage of Americans who reported experiencing "great stress" at least once a week increased from 55 percent to 64 percent. Nearly one third of Americans, especially women, adults in their 40s, and those with a four-year college degree, felt "great stress" almost every day. Although many Americans experience high levels of stress, 65 percent reported that they "consciously take steps to control or reduce the stress."

Stress Management Principles

Much has been written about controlling stress, and the suggestions can be summarized in five basic stress management methods:

1. Control Stressors

Stressors are everywhere, and this stress management principle is based on the idea that you have the power to diminish, modify, or eliminate as many stressors as you need to to accomplish your goals. For example, if you are going to climb a mountain, you can make the trip miserable by hiking too fast with a very heavy backpack, or satisfying and pleasurable by walking at a moderate pace with a lighter load. Same goal, same path, but different loads and tempos.

Let's say a college student is taking a heavy academic load in a subject area that is too difficult for him (biochemistry), working 15 hours a week to help pay for expenses, living in a crowded and noisy apartment with an unbearable roommate, experiencing constant transportation problems because of a car that keeps breaking down, and having to deal with crushing family problems because of the divorce of his parents. The first step would be for the student to sit down, make a list of all his major goals, in order of importance, and then catalog each of the stressors along with plans either to eliminate or to modify them.

For example, because finishing biochemistry is necessary for him to achieve his major life goal of becoming a physician, he may increase his study time by quitting work and taking out a loan. He could move closer to campus, try to find more desirable living accommodations, and walk or bicycle for transportation until finances improve.

Stressors can be managed by controlling the pace of life and the load carried. A key is to avoid crowding too much into the schedule, and learning to control circumstances until the pace of life is suitable to your psychological makeup. Control your circumstances—don't let them control you.

2. Let Your Mind Choose the Reaction

This strategy is also called "stress reaction management." We already mentioned that when a stress reaction takes place in the body (the fight-or-flight response), various stress hormones increase, depressing immune function, increasing blood pressure, etc. This response has a negative effect on a person's health, so the goal is to avoid letting the stress reaction take place.

One fundamental principle of the way you are designed is that when stressful events happen, they have to be seen, heard, felt, or sensed by the brain one way or the other. Then the mind interprets the event, and a reaction takes place. The good news is that when a stressor presents itself, you can decide what reaction will take place. The bad news is that we often have knee-jerk reactions to various stressful events without allowing the mind to reason them out calmly. In other words, humans are largely responsible for creating their own emotional reactions and disturbances—reactions that can be controlled.

Marcus Aurelius stated long ago, "If you are distressed by anything external, the pain is not due to the thing itself but to your estimate of it. This you have the power to revoke at any time."

So when an event takes place (e.g., a flat tire on your way to work), you can choose how you will react, either letting the stress response rise up within you (as you kick the tire and grimace in anger) with all of its health-destroying effects, or taking a calmer and more reasoned approach (I'll call at the first opportunity and work it out with the boss).

3. Seek the Social Support of Others

A survey of a cross section of the American population has shown that as many as one fourth, especially divorced parents, single mothers, persons never married, and housewives, feel extremely lonely at some time during any given month (*American Journal of Health Promotion* 4, No. 1 [1989]: 18-31).

Studies have now demonstrated that when people are socially isolated (few social interactions, contacts, and relationships with family and friends, neighbors or the "society at large"), they are more vulnerable to sickness, mental stress, and even early death.

In one nine-year study of 7,000 residents of Alameda County, California, study subjects with few ties to other people had death rates from various diseases two to five times higher than those with more associations. The researchers measured social ties by looking at whether or not they were married, the number of close friends and relatives they had, and how often they were in contact with them, church attendance and involvement in informal and formal groups (*American Journal of Epidemiology* 109 [1979]: 186-204). Social support means reaching out to other people, sharing emotional, social, physical, financial, and other types of comfort and assistance.

The Institute of Medicine, Division of Health Promotion and Disease Prevention, recently published its landmark book entitled *The Second Fifty Years: Promoting Health and Preventing Disability* (Washington, D.C.: National Academy Press, 1990). In this document, the institute concluded that "a lack of family and community supports plays an important role in the development of disease. An absence of social support weakens the body's defenses through psychological stress. Isolated individuals must be identified, and strategies for increasing social contact and diminishing feelings of loneliness must be developed.

Clinicians, family, friends, and social institutions bear a responsibility for diminishing social isolation.''

Solomon had much to say on this topic, promoting the concept that each of us can improve the health and cheer of our fellows. ''An anxious heart weighs a man down, but a kind word cheers him up'' (Proverbs 12:25, NIV). ''The tongue that brings healing is a tree of life'' (Proverbs 15:4, NIV). ''A cheerful look brings joy to the heart, and good news gives health to the bones'' (verse 30, NIV). ''Pleasant words are a honeycomb, sweet to the soul and healing to the bones'' (Proverbs 16:24, NIV).

4. Keep Healthy

When the body is healthy from adequate exercise, sleep, food, fresh air and sunshine, water, and relaxation, stressors can be better handled.

Regular exercise is one of the most important habits in this regard. Notes Dr. John Farquhar of Stanford University, ''Through prudent, regular, and systematic use of your body, you will discover a greater sense of well-being, far greater energy, and a calmer, more relaxed attitude toward the pressures you experience daily.'' In chapter 11, we will review evidence from studies that have shown that depression, anxiety, and mental stress can each be diminished while psychological well-being and feelings of vigor are improved through regular physical activity.

Sleep problems have become a modern epidemic, taking an enormous toll on our bodies and minds. Desperately trying to fit more into the day, many people are stealing extra hours from the night. The result, say sleep researchers, is a sleep deficit that undermines health, sabotages productivity, blackens mood, clouds judgment, and increases the risk of accidents (Better Sleep Council, P.O. Box 13, Washington, D.C. 20044).

Yet even those who want to sleep more often can't. In recent surveys, half of men and women say they've had trouble sleeping. The Better Sleep Council gives a number of guidelines for improving sleep, including: (1) keep regular sleeping hours; (2) exercise regularly; (3) cut down on stimulants (coffee, tea, cola drinks, chocolate); (4) sleep on a good bed; (5) don't smoke (nicotine is a stronger stimulant than caffeine); (6) go for quality, not just quantity; (7) set aside a worry or planning time early in the evening; (8) don't go to bed stuffed or starved; (9) develop a sleep ritual.

5. Love God and Serve Others

Solomon promoted the idea that "he who refreshes others will himself be refreshed" (Proverbs 11:25, NIV). This concept has been echoed by many others, including Dr. Albert Schweitzer, who once wrote, "I don't know what your destiny will be. But I do know that the only ones among you who will find true happiness are those who find a place to serve."

Dr. Hans Selye echoed this thought in his book *Stress Without Distress* (New York: New American Library, 1974): "My own code is based on the view that to achieve peace of mind and fulfillment through self-expression, most men need a commitment to work in the service of some cause that they can respect."

Keep in mind that the most important strategy of all is the maintenance of a close relationship with God our Creator and Redeemer. The Bible is rich in promises of health, peace, and satisfaction for those who place their trust and love in God.

"Cast all your anxiety on him because he cares for you" (1 Peter 5:7, NIV). "Do not be anxious about anything, but in everything, by prayer and petition, with thanksgiving, present your requests to God. And the peace of God, which transcends all understanding, will guard your hearts and your minds in Christ Jesus" (Philippians 4:6, 7, NIV).

Christ, as the "Prince of Peace" (Isaiah 9:6), is the only means by which we can have peace with ourselves, others, and God. And no matter what the circumstance, He is always there as a buffer against the many stressors of this life.

"For I am convinced that neither death nor life, neither angels nor demons, neither the present nor the future, nor any powers, neither height nor depth, nor anything else in all creation, will be able to separate us from the love of God that is in Christ Jesus our Lord" (Romans 8:38, 39, NIV).

CHAPTER 11

The Mind and Health

"It is not a soul, it is not a body that we are training up; it is a man, and we ought not to divide him into two parts."—Montaigne.

Perhaps the most dramatic example in Scripture of the influence that the mind can have on the body is the experience of Christ during His last hours before His death. From the Garden of Gethsemane to His final words on the cross, "It is finished," (John 19:30), we see Christ suffering mental stress as no man has or ever will.

"Christ was the prince of sufferers; but His suffering was from a sense of the malignity of sin. . . . The Saviour could not see through the portals of the tomb. . . . He feared that sin was so offensive to God that Their separation was to be eternal." That cry, uttered 'with a loud voice' (Matthew 27:50; Luke 23:46), at the moment of death, the stream of blood and water that flowed from His side, declared that He died of a broken heart. His heart was broken by mental anguish" (*The Desire of Ages*, pp. 752, 753, 772).

In a highly unusual article in the prestigious *Journal of the American Medical Association*, a group of medical doctors from the Mayo Clinic in Rochester, Minnesota, recently described, from a medical viewpoint, their interpretation of the physical death of Jesus Christ (255 [1986]: 1455-1463).

The clinicians carefully interpreted the physical aspects

103

surrounding Christ's death, including His bloody sweat in the Garden of Gethsemane, and intimate details on the medical effects of scourging and crucifixion practices. They concluded that the bloody sweat was evidence that Christ was in a highly emotional state, and that He died from this and other multiple causes including shock from blood loss, failure to breathe as a result of exhaustion while on the cross, and perhaps acute heart failure.

In the words of these medical doctors: "The severe scourging, with its intense pain and appreciable blood loss, most probably left Jesus in a preshock state. The physical and mental abuse meted out by the Jews and the Romans, as well as the lack of food, water, and sleep, also contributed to His generally weakened state. Therefore, even before the actual crucifixion, Jesus' physical condition was at least serious and possibly critical. . . . The major pathophysiologic effect of crucifixion, beyond the excruciating pain, was a marked interference with normal respiration. . . . A fatal cardiac arrhythmia may have accounted for the apparent catastrophic terminal event."

The Relationship Between the Mind and Health

A growing number of medical journals are devoting more attention to the view that mental states can have a profound effect on a person's physical health. Studies have shown that being chronically anxious, depressed, or emotionally distressed is associated with deterioration of health.

For example, in one study of 1,300 graduates of the Johns Hopkins Medical School, depression was found to be an important predictor of heart disease. In England, heart disease was more likely to develop in people who had chronic mild anxiety and depression than in those who did not. In a study of 10,000 Israeli men, anxiety over problems and conflicts in areas of finance, family, and coworkers was associated with two to three times the risk for development of heart disease.

In a 17-year study of 2,000 middle-aged men, depression was associated with twice the risk of death from cancer. In a one-year study of 100 people, flus and colds were four times as likely to occur following stressful life events. In Australia, the number of days with flu and cold symptoms were double in high versus low-stressed individuals.

Dr. Donald Girard, from the Oregon Health Sciences University, has reviewed the literature on this subject and concluded that repressed feelings of loss, denial, depression, inflexibility, conformity, lack of social ties, high levels of anxiety and dissatisfaction, and many life-changing events are associated with increased cancers, heart disease, and infection (*Western Journal of Medicine* 142 [1985]: 358-363). Writes Dr. Girard, "It seems that the best advice the physician can offer patients is that good mental health is important for maintaining physical well-being."

National surveys suggest that marital happiness contributes far more to global happiness than any other variable, including satisfaction with work and friendships. Survey results indicate that divorced and separated individuals have poorer mental and physical health than married, widowed, or single adults. Marital disruption has been found to be the single most powerful predictor of stress-related physical illness, with separated individuals having about 30 percent more acute illnesses and physician visits than married adults. Depression of immune function has been associated with marital discord.

A number of other studies have found bereavement and a lack of social and community ties to be associated with an overall increase in mortality. In a study of 95,647 widowed individuals, mortality during the first week following widowhood was more than twofold compared to expected rates, especially from cardiovascular disease, violent causes, and suicides.

Dr. William Ruberman of New York has reported that heart disease patients classified as being socially isolated (few contacts with friends, relatives, church or club groups) and having a high degree of life stress had more than four times the risk of dying from heart disease as men with low levels of isolation and stress. This supports the statement made by William Harvey in 1628:

"Every affection of the mind that is attended with either pain or pleasure, hope or fear, is the cause of an agitation whose influence extends to the heart."

Dr. George Vaillant of Harvard University followed the 40-year history of 204 men and found that poor mental health was associated with increased disease and death over and above the effects of drug abuse, obesity, or family history of long life. Concluded Vaillant, "Good mental health facilitates our survival."

Mental Anxiety and Depression in the U.S.

In the United States, 19 percent of the population is affected by one or more mental disorders during any given six-month period. The direct cost of mental health care in the United States is more than $22 billion per year. Anxiety disorders are the most prevalent of all mental illnesses. Depression is also fairly common among Americans, afflicting between 9 percent and 20 percent during any given month.

Recently the U.S. Public Health Service conducted the National Health Interview Survey that included questions on the amount of stress experienced in the past two weeks and the effect of stress on health. About half of U.S. adults reported experiencing at least a moderate amount of stress in the two weeks preceding the date of interview. Individuals with higher education and income levels were more likely to feel that they experienced stress than those with lower education and income.

Despite this relatively high prevalence of stress in the population, only 11 percent of adults had sought help in the past year for a personal or emotional problem. Obviously a large percentage of the population could be benefited by various stress management techniques.

Exercise and the Mind

"Keep the body in strength and vigor so that it may be able to obey and execute the orders of the mind" (John Locke).

We have seen that poor mental health is associated with poor physical health. Is there proof for the converse association? Is a healthy and fit body related to psychological health? Were the ancient Greeks right in their assertion that a physically fit and strong body would lead to a sound mind?

The part of the brain that enables us to exercise, the motor cortex, lies only a few millimeters away from the part of the brain strata that deals with thought and feeling. Might their proximity mean that when exercise stimulates the motor cortex, it has a parallel effect on cognition and emotion?

Since the beginning of time many have believed in the "cerebral satisfaction" of exercise. The Greeks maintained that exercise made their minds more lucid. Aristotle started his peripatetic school in 335 B.C. The school was so named because of Aristotle's habit of walking up and down (peripaton) the paths of the Lyceum in Athens while thinking or lecturing to his students who walked with him. Plato and Socrates had also practiced the art of peripatetics, as did later the Roman *Ordo Vagorum*, or walking scholars. Centuries later, Oliver Wendell Holmes explained that "in walking the will and the muscles are so accustomed to working together and perform their task with so little expenditure of force that the intellect is left comparatively free."

John F. Kennedy echoed the Greek ideal when he said, "Physical fitness is not only one of the most important keys to a healthy body; it is the basis of dynamic and creative intellectual activity. Intelligence and skill can only function at the peak of their capacity when the body is strong. Hardy spirits and tough minds usually inhabit sound bodies."

The highly acclaimed Perrier Survey of Fitness in America, conducted by Louis Harris and Associates, showed that modern-day men and women believe in the Greek concept of a "strong mind in a strong body." The survey found that those who have a deep commitment to exercise reported feeling more relaxed, less tired, and more disciplined, a sense of looking better, greater self-confidence, greater productivity in work, and in general, more of being at one with themselves.

Researchers have been eager to study the belief that physical activity improves psychological health. Thousands of studies have now been conducted investigating whether or not exercise really results in measurable improvements in depression, anxiety, intelligence, self-concept, and other psychological parameters. Exciting new data support this relationship.

Recently Dr. Tom Stephens of Canada directed the evaluation of data from four national surveys in the U.S. and Canada. "The inescapable conclusion from these four national studies," says Dr. Stephens, "is that physical activity is positively associated with good mental health, especially positive mood, general well-being, and less anxiety and depression." This relationship was found to be stronger for the older age group (+40 years of age) than for the younger, and for women than for men.

During the past 25 years, a large number of studies have shown that life events of all types (marriage, divorce, buying a house, losing a job, moving, surgery, etc.) are significant stressors, leading to predictable physical and psychologic health problems. Several recent studies have shown, however, that such life stress has less negative impact on the health of physically active individuals.

For example, in a four-year study of 278 managers from 12 different corporations, physical activity was found to have a buffering effect on the relationship between life events and illness. In other words, corporate managers who were active experienced less health problems from the stress they experienced than did inactive managers. Because it is not always practical or even possible to avoid many stressful life events, regular aerobic exercise may be one way to reduce the impact of stress on health.

Many other studies have indicated the value of physical activity for improved psychological health. A team of researchers at Duke University showed that after 10 weeks of walking and jogging 135 minutes a week, exercising adults experienced decreased anxiety, depression, and fatigue, with elevated vigor. Dr. Carlyle Folkins of the University of California at Davis has shown that regular exercise by policemen and firemen is associated with decreased anxiety and depression. Dr. John Griest of the University of Wisconsin compared the effects of a running program against psychotherapy with depressed subjects. Running was found to be at least as effective as psychotherapy in alleviating moderate depression. A study at Loma Linda University showed that three miles of brisk walking, five days a week, dramatically increased psychological well-being while decreasing anxiety after just six weeks compared to a sedentary control group.

Results from some studies have suggested that short-term memory and intellectual function may be improved during or shortly after exercise. In one study, subjects exercising moderately on a stationary bicycle demonstrated an increase in short-term memory, comprehension, and ability to react mentally during the exercise bout.

The Greeks, who walked while discussing topics of importance, were believers in the ability of exercise to improve mental function. More research is needed to study the long-term impact of regular physical exercise on mental cognition during nonexercise time periods.

How Exercise Helps the Mind

Just how and why exercise improves psychological health is at this time still unresolved. Some of the theories involve the effects of exercise on various hormones and other body chemicals.

The body has an amazing, recently discovered hormonal system of morphine-like chemicals called endogenous opioids. These hormones are of interest because their receptors are found in the areas of the brain associated with emotion, pleasure, pain, and behavior. During exercise, the pituitary increases its production of beta-endorphin, one of the endogenous opioids, with the result that its concentration rises in the blood. It also appears that levels of beta-endorphin rise in the brain during exercise, helping the person feel better.

Exercise may also enhance the activity of special chemicals

in the brain called neurotransmitters. Dr. Charles Ransford of Hillsdale College in Michigan has reviewed the data in this area, and although much more study is needed, he speculates that exercise may alter levels of norepinephrine, dopamine, and serotonin in the brain, decreasing depression.

Dr. James Wiese of Alberta Hospital and a research team at Arizona State University have both discovered that during exercise there is an increase in brain emission of alpha waves. These brainwaves are associated with a relaxed, meditation-like state, and appear 20 minutes into a 30-minute exercise bout, and are still measurable after the exercise is over. Researchers speculate that the increased alpha wave power could contribute to the psychological benefits of exercise, including reductions in anxiety and depression.

Other researchers suggest that exercise decreases muscle electrical tension. Some advance the idea that exercise increases oxygen transport to the brain. During exercise, deep body temperature is increased, which may decrease muscle tension and influence certain brain neurotransmitters.

Practical Implications

One of the amazing facts to come out of the research presented in this chapter is that the same amount of exercise that helps the heart also helps the brain. The American College of Sports Medicine has established that 30 to 60 minutes of moderate exercise, several days a week, is essential for both health and fitness. Most of the studies mentioned in this chapter used the same exercise criteria, showing that as the heart is strengthened, so is the brain.

With exercise, we have a strong weapon to help counter the never-ending onslaught of stress, anxiety, and depression associated with our modern era. Exercise can act as a buffer, decreasing the strain of stressful events, while alleviating anxiety and depression, and elevating mood.

The decrease in anxiety and depression, and the elevation in mood that comes with regular exercise, should help "brain-workers'' feel better during their work. What this means for busy students and workers everywhere is that time spent in exercise may not be lost. Instead, the half-hour exercise session could mean enhanced mental functioning and greater time efficiency. Including exercise breaks for normally sedentary office workers or students may actually enhance productivity of work and study.

CHAPTER 12

Aging Healthfully and Gracefully

"How old would you be if you didn't know how old you were?"—Satchel Paige.

What is the potential for human longevity? What sort of vitality can we have in later life? Is it possible, as the Bible says, to "come to the grave in full vigor, like sheaves gathered in season" (Job 5:26, NIV)?

Newspapers in Oakland, California, recently reported the death of local resident Arthur Reed, age 124. In Japan, Shigechiyo Isumi died in 1986 in his 121st year. Dr. Walter Bortz in his book *We Live Too Short and Die Too Long* states there is enough evidence to support the idea that humans today are capable of living to the age of 120, or about 1 million hours. This is much higher than the average 75 years that Americans can expect to live.

The Senior Citizen Explosion

Length of life has increased remarkably during the twentieth century. Life expectancy at birth (the number of years a newborn baby can expect to live) reached a new high of 75 years in 1990, much higher than the 47 years recorded for those living in the year 1900. Increases in life expectancy at birth during the first half of this century occurred mainly because the number of babies who died decreased dramatically. More Americans survived to middle age. By contrast, increases in longevity in recent years have largely resulted from lower death rates from heart disease and stroke among the middle-aged and elderly.

The fastest-growing minority in the United States today is the elderly—those who reach or pass the age of 65. Nearly 30 million elderly persons live in the U.S., a number that is expected to climb to 64.6 million, or 21 percent of the total population, by the year 2030. The baby boom is being replaced by the senior citizen explosion, with the 65 and over group growing twice as fast as the rest of the population.

It is difficult to comprehend that in 1900 only 25 percent of individuals in the U.S. lived beyond age 65, while in 1985 approximately 70 percent survived age 65, and 30 percent lived to be 80 or more. If present trends continue, within the next 10 or 20 years almost half of deaths will occur after age 80.

Within the past five years, intense interest has focused on those 85 years and older (termed the "very old"). This group is expected to be the most rapidly growing population segment for the next 25 years, with a projected increase from 2.7 million in 1985 to approximately 7 million by the year 2015.

Although these trends are exciting, concern has been expressed by some leaders regarding the quality of life. Experts say that quality of life is not keeping pace with increases in quantity of life. The majority of elderly people have at least one major type of disease with multiple health problems. Half of the elderly have arthritis, two thirds have high blood pressure, 30 percent have a hearing impairment, and 26 percent have heart disease. Heart disease and cancer account for three fourths of all deaths among the elderly. Osteoporosis, defined as a decrease in the amount of bone leading to fractures, is present in a large number of the elderly. By the year 2000 it is estimated that 3.8 million elderly people will have senile dementia, especially Alzheimer's disease.

The Aging Process

Aging refers to the normal yet irreversible changes that occur in the body during one's lifetime. The aging process occurs in all people, but for those over 65 years of age, it often results in significant changes in quality of life.

George Burns once quipped, "You'll know you're old when everything hurts and what doesn't hurt doesn't work; when you get winded playing chess; when you stoop to tie your shoelaces and ask yourself, 'What else can I do while I'm down here?'; when everybody goes to your birthday party and stands around the cake just to get warm."

What factors are responsible for the aging process that leads to death in humans? There are two major theories of aging. "Error" theories speculate that with advancing age, we become less able to repair damage caused by malfunctions inside the body or damage imposed from outside the body. For example, chemical and hormone changes that occur with aging, and a less effective immune system may finally lead to death. The body may be less able to combat infection or destroy abnormal body cells. "Program" theories of aging suggest that an internal clock starts ticking at conception and is programmed to run just so long. Some researchers feel that human body cells can only divide a certain number of times until stopping, leading to death.

As a person ages, some of the changes that take place in the body include a decrease in ability to taste, smell, hear, and see; loss of teeth and bone mass in the jaw area; decrease in ability to digest and absorb food; reduction in muscle and bone mass throughout the body; impairment of memory, judgment, feelings, personality, and ability to speak; decrease in reaction time and ability to balance, diminished liver and kidney function; and a decrease in heart and lung fitness.

Interestingly, many of the changes that accompany aging are of the same type that can be expected with inactivity. In fact, much of the deterioration attributed to aging can be explained by the fact that people tend to exercise less as they age. All living cells, tissues, and organs start to age when their particular activity is impaired, and the body as a whole will age faster without regular exercise.

Hippocrates, the ancient Greek physician, observed this long ago: "All parts of the body which have a function, if used in moderation and exercised in labors in which each is accustomed, become thereby healthy and well-developed, and age more slowly, but if unused and left idle, they become liable to disease, defective in growth, and age quickly."

Researchers have now shown that there is a big difference in the quality of life among the elderly. Many, because of optimal lifestyles, are living active, independent lives into their ninth and tenth decades. The difference for many is a matter of choice.

Hulda Crooks and Mavis Lindgren are two remarkable Seventh-day Adventist women reaping the benefits of wise lifestyle choices. Their lives are centered in their Creator and balanced by simple, healthful habits such as good nutrition, plenty of outdoor activity, sufficient rest, avoidance of harmful substances, and gratitude of heart. Hulda turned 95, and Mavis 85, years of age in 1992. Hulda climbs mountains, Mavis runs marathons. Both discovered in their 50s and 60s that vitality belongs not only to the young but to the young at heart. And both women believe in the importance of spiritual health to overall health.

Grandma Whitney

Hulda was born and raised on a Canadian farm, where she grew up on a diet of meat, milk, cream, butter, eggs, and plenty of vigorous physical activity. In her father's country store, she had free access as well to a large barrel of hard candy at one end of the counter and soft-centered chocolates at the other. By age 16, at a height of only five feet six inches, she weighed 160 pounds despite her physical activity. At 18, having completed only five grades of country schooling, she joined the Seventh-day Adventist Church.

Adopting the SDA health philosophy, Hulda became a lacto-ovovegetarian. For more than 75 years she has followed this diet, which has had much to do with her present vitality. She eats a wide variety of fruits, vegetables, whole grains, and nuts, with a moderate amount of low-fat milk and a few eggs. A computerized analysis of her diet showed more than half of the nutrients coming from carbohydrates (59 percent carbohydrates, 25 percent fat), with vitamins A, C, and E at two to three times the recommended level. Some are surprised that she has such an excellent nutrient breakdown without the use of any supplements. However, as Hulda maintains, "I don't think I need them. I have an abundance of fresh fruits and vegetables as well as the cooked kind. I don't think I need extra vitamins. I believe we can take too many vitamins and the body then has the job of throwing out the excess." All reputable nutrition experts agree with her.

Hulda completed her dietetics training at Loma Linda University in 1927 (also spending some time at Pacific Union College), but not without some expense to her health. Despite her newly acquired education, Hulda admits, "I wasn't worth much. I was nervous and perpetually tired." It was then that she began to implement a truly balanced yet simple lifestyle. When it comes to diet and exercise, Hulda says, "You can't separate the two. You need both a good diet and sufficient exercise. The diet of course provides the materials for the body's functions. The exercise is absolutely essential in keeping up a good circulation. If we don't exercise, the circulation is sluggish and that affects the entire body, the mental as well as the rest of the body."

It was a thoughtful and farsighted husband, Samuel A. Crooks, M.D., who encouraged her love for the outdoors and discouraged her spending long hours in the kitchen. He knew the element in which she was most happy—nature—and fostered that love by buying her lots of nature study books.

Sam had a heart condition that prevented him from climbing high mountains. Still, he urged Hulda to walk with other hikers. "One summer," Hulda recounts, "while we were driving in the vicinity of Lone Pine, California, Sam pointed out the window. 'See that peak?' My eyes followed his direction. 'That's Mount Whitney, the highest mountain in the continental United States,' he informed me. It looked awesome." Little did either of them guess that nearly 30 years later Hulda would climb that mountain.

After a coronary attack took Sam in the fall of 1950, Hulda's spiritual faith and the object lessons she found in nature provided a tranquilizer for her emotions. She says, "Nature is the picture book of the Bible. . . . When I started climbing the mountains, I saw how the trees adjusted to the rising altitude and increasing severity of the elements. This made a very deep impression on my mind in a time when I was under very great emotional stress after my husband died."

In 1962, at age 66, encouraged by her friends, Hulda climbed Mount Whitney (14,495 feet) for the first time. At age 70 she began jogging (at first in her backyard) to give her improved heart and lung fitness for the strenuous climb. Training year-round for her annual Mount Whitney climb, Hulda, now in her mid-90s, has conquered the mountain 23 times. She has also hiked the entire 212 miles of the John Muir trail, and just since she turned 81, has climbed 88 of the highest peaks in southern California, including Mount San Gorgonio (11,500 feet).

During the past several years Hulda has replaced jogging with walking (in her ninetieth year she walked 1,200 miles). In June and July, before her August attempts on Mount Whitney, she intensifies her training, climbing stairs and hills. "The reason I stopped jogging is that it is easier to fall when you jog." Hulda believes the benefits of walking are equal to those of jogging. "It takes a little longer, especially if you can jog faster like young people can. They can do it much faster that way, but I don't recommend jogging for older people unless they feel safe in doing it."

Using a sophisticated computerized system in the Human Performance Laboratory at Loma Linda University, Hulda's VO_2 max was measured. VO_2 max is the ability of the body to use oxygen during heavy exercise. It is the best criterion of a person's overall physical fitness level. At age 90 Hulda's results showed that she had a VO_2 max equivalent to that of a woman 30 years younger. Amazingly, after two hard months of hill and stair climbing, Hulda improved her VO$_2$ max by 7 percent, demonstrating that even 90-year-old women can improve their physical fitness.

Hulda's body fat just before her Mount Whitney climb was 25 percent, that of a college woman. Her HDL cholesterol was 53 mg./dl., giving her a total cholesterol/HDL cholesterol ratio of 4.2, prepresenting below average risk of heart disease.

When asked if there are days when she just doesn't feel like exercising or going for a walk, Hulda replied, "Usually I do it anyway." In agreement with the late Dr. Paul D. White, President Eisenhower's world-famous heart specialist, in his book *The Brain Is on Top,* Hulda says, "If the brain is on top, it should be in charge and tell the rest of the body what to do. And so that's what I do. Once in a while I don't go out if there's some special reason, but usually I go out. Six days a week anyway. . . . I think it is my responsibility to take care of my body. Personal health maintenance is what is being urged on people now. If I don't take care of my body, nobody will. And so, I just feel it is my privilege and my pleasure and my responsibility to care for the body that the Lord gave me."

"Grandma Whitney," as she is dubbed by the press here and abroad, is known for her captivating stories both along the climb and at the top. In 1986 she spoke to a crowd of 50 near the top of Mount Whitney. "As people, we have bodies that we must take care of. Watch what you eat. Get your exercise. We are also beings with spiritual bodies that we must take care of. Climbing a mountain can help you with your spiritual body, if you let it." Congressman Jerry Lewis, one of those in the group, said, "If she didn't walk one more step, she will have succeeded beyond any reasonable person's wildest imagination."

In 1987, Dentsu Inc., Japan's largest advertising firm, thought it a novel idea to have a 91-year-old woman climb with them in celebration of the 60th anniversary of the Dentsu employees' annual climb of Mount Fuji. Hulda was sent by Loma Linda's Mayor Elmer Digneo as an "ambassador of goodwill and healthful living."

A good friend and primary coordinator of the event, Dr. Bill Andress, accompanied Hulda (who walked unaided) the entire 12,389 feet up Japan's highest peak along with Dentsu representatives and Dr. Hongo of the Tokyo Adventist Hospital.

On July 24, 1987, Hulda watched the sun rise from the top of Mount Fuji. Six weeks later she was on top of Mount Whitney once again. Hulda became the oldest woman in the history of Japan to climb Mount Fuji and the oldest person, man or woman, to climb Mount Whitney. These back-to-back achievements caught the attention of the world press, and Hulda's story was told and retold in the media from China to the United States.

Hulda's achievements, as laboratory tests have proved, are not because of unique genetic endowment. Instead, they are the result of proper health stewardship—lifestyle rooted in a deep faith in God and balanced by regular exercise, sufficient rest, and a vegetarian diet. The vitality of Hulda Crooks is within the reach of most people who make the same choice of lifestyle.

Hulda's special message to the young is "Look ahead!" To the young, old age seems a long way off, but it is never too soon to begin a balanced lifestyle. The benefits gained by an improved lifestyle are not only investments in the future, but dividends to be experienced today. For the same reason, people of all ages should realize that it is never too late to begin.

Hulda encourages those who would like to start an exercise program to first "make up their minds to do it. It's not easy to really make up your mind and think that you have time to do it. You find time, and as you work at it, it becomes part of your program. The best thing to do is to start gradually and to increase your effort. Dr. Paul W. White also made this statement: 'The best way to keep fit is to walk and walk and walk.' And that's my type of exercise."

Amazing Mavis

Mavis Lindgren stands only five feet two inches and weighs just 102 pounds, but this 85-year-old nurse is big on achievement. Called "Amazing Mavis" by *Sports Illustrated* and many of her admirers, Mavis Lindgren holds many national and world age-group records for running events from the 10-kilometer to the 26.2-mile marathon.

Mavis is a true late-bloomer, having overcome an unhealthy past. As a child in Canada she suffered whooping cough and pneumonia, which weakened her lungs. As an adult she experienced annual bouts of severe bronchitis.

It wasn't until her early 60s, after listening to a lecture by Loma Linda University professor Dr. Charles Thomas, that Mavis was inspired to take responsibility for her health. Hoping and praying that exercise might help cure her worsening lungs, Mavis began walking faithfully every day.

In the beginning the walks were short. Decades of inactivity had added 20 extra pounds of body fat plus weakened her heart and skeletal muscles. Slowly she increased her walking distance, and after several weeks began adding jogging steps to her exercise routine.

As the months rolled by, Mavis experienced a rebirth of health. She lost the 20 extra pounds and was gratified and overjoyed to discover that her lung problem had also disappeared. "I haven't been sick a day since then," she often states. Those first few faltering steps marked the end of a lifetime of illness.

As walking became easier, Mavis discovered that she also loved to run. After a long period of adjustment, she found herself running five miles, six days a week, and enjoying it. She maintained this regimen for several years.

When Mavis was 70, the running world discovered her, thanks in great part to the persuasiveness of her son, a medical doctor who realized her unusual potential and signed her up for the Avenue of the Giants Marathon. Training more than 50 miles a week in preparation for her first marathon, Mavis successfully finished the 26.2-mile event, setting an age-group world record.

Since then, Mavis has raced in 60 full marathons, resetting the world record four times (her fastest time is 4 hours and 34 minutes). In the fall of 1984, she also established a world best time for women over the age of 70 in the 10-kilometer (6.2-mile) event, racing to a 57-minute, 34-second finish. Mavis also became the oldest woman to run the race to the top of Pikes Peak in Colorado. She is always quick to remind, however, that she really only races against herself—she is not a competitor. There are times when she is the only person running in her age group.

Mavis, a petite, modest woman, has been the object of much attention from the press, yet she continually directs the limelight away from herself and toward God. She has a busy traveling schedule, flying to all parts of the United States, Canada, and the Caribbean, but still keeps up with her demanding training schedule, which averages 50 miles of running per week.

Mavis maximizes her training by eating a high carbohydrate, vegetarian diet that helps restore her muscle glycogen levels for the next training bout.

As mentioned earlier, the best measure of heart, lung, and blood vessel fitness is the VO_2 max. Mavis' test results showed her to have a VO_2 max equivalent to the fitness of the average college woman. In other words, Mavis has the heart and lungs of a woman 58 years younger!

Body composition testing also showed that Mavis is only 12 percent body fat. To put this in perspective, the average college woman is 25 percent body fat, and the average middle-aged woman is 32 percent body fat.

Other results showed that Mavis has a breathing capacity 40 percent above what is predicted for women her age, an amazing statistic in light of her former lung problems. Each time she is reminded of her exceptional fitness level she exclaims, "I just thank God for all the health He's given me."

Mavis is still training hard, traveling far and wide as she participates in running events. She enjoys the tough challenge of running through the wooded hills surrounding her northern California home. As a Seventh-day Adventist Christian, Mavis plans to continue running as long as God gives her strength. "I look upon my running as a means to help others improve their own lifestyles and better glorify God."

The story of Mavis is particularly compelling in that she appears to be defeating Old Man Time. Once an elderly, overweight woman with lung problems, she seemingly threw off the limitations common to age, and ran her way back to the "fountain of youth." Although the process of aging finally takes over in every person, Mavis has shown that it is possible to maintain an extremely high level of fitness even into the twilight years.

It's Your Choice

We have every reason to believe that a high quality of life in old age is possible for many who make the same lifestyle decisions that Hulda and Mavis have made—trust in God, regular exercise and rest, a healthful diet, and abstinence from cigarettes, alcohol, and other drugs. The big message they bring is it's never too late to start.

Limitations are but misperceptions, for, "as it is written: 'No eye has seen, no ear has heard, no mind has conceived what God has prepared for those who love him' " (1 Corinthians 2:9, NIV). The stories of Mavis Lindgren and Hulda Crooks give hope to the millions who today seek a more vibrant life during their sojourn on this earth.

CHAPTER 13

Health Promotion
in Your Church

"Health promotion is the science and art of helping people change their lifestyle to move toward a state of optimal health. Optimal health is defined as a balance of physical, emotional, social, spiritual and intellectual health." —
Michael O'Donnell, Editor,
American Journal of Health Promotion.

In chapter 4 the process of health behavior change was described, along with practical steps to achieve change. This chapter reviews the process of health promotion and includes practical ideas for your church health program. Seventh-day Adventists have traditionally connected health programs with community outreach. How can churches participate in this work more effectively?

The Meaning of Health Promotion

In 1979 the surgeon general's report on health promotion and disease prevention, *Healthy People*, was published. This was a landmark document that signaled America's needed determination to do battle against heart disease, stroke, cancer, diabetes, and the other leading killers of the Western world. Citing poor diets, lack of exercise, obesity, cigarette smoking, alcoholism, and drug abuse as the major lifestyle causes of these diseases, Americans were given the challenge to bear more responsibility for their personal habits.

However, changing the health practices of Americans has proved to be more difficult than once hoped (see chapter 4). As a result, scores of researchers throughout the United States have turned their attention to defining better how health can be effectively promoted in the community.

As stated in the quote at the beginning of this chapter, the health promotion process seeks to help people change their lifestyles so that they can enjoy better physical, mental, social, and spiritual health.

Dr. Lawrence Green, one of America's foremost experts on health promotion, gives this definition: "Health promotion is the combination of educational and environmental supports for actions and conditions of living conducive to health" (*Health Promotion Planning: An Educational and Environmental Approach* [Mountain View, Calif.: Mayfield Publishing Company, 1991]).

The purpose of health promotion is to help people gain better control of the factors that determine their health. In order for this to be achieved, an optimum mix of responsibility should be shared between individuals, families, health professionals, churches and volunteer agencies, private or governmental organizations, and local or national agencies.

Sometimes community health can be improved when laws are passed prohibiting smoking in public places, or the American Heart Association uses the media to raise public awareness of the need to reduce fat in the diet, or the federal government places a higher tax on alcoholic beverages, or the local church conducts a blood pressure screening program. Promotion of health in the community is easier when people work together in an organized fashion, and a supportive social environment is created.

A Plan for Health Promotion in Your Church

Here are seven steps recommended for each church seeking to improve the health of its community.

Step 1—Choose or hire a health professional or other individual with appropriate training to lead out in the health outreach program of the church. This cannot be emphasized enough—everything depends on qualified leadership. A health committee can then be formed to help with planning.

Step 2—Network with pertinent health organizations and individuals in the community. Many organizations are eager to share expertise and materials, and to cooperate with local churches in their health promotion programs. Community health leaders can also give invaluable guidance regarding the most significant health problems in the local community.

Health promotion programs will be much more effective if they are part of a comprehensive community plan. For example, if the church finds that blood pressure screening programs are already ongoing and meeting the needs of the community, other screening programs can be developed and implemented to avoid overlap.

Step 3—Determine the resources available to develop and implement screening programs and other health programs. These include personnel, equipment, facilities, and finances. For example, if the church decides that it would like to conduct a computerized screening program in the community, several organizational details will need to be worked out, including the computer and software, money to purchase these items, people to run the programs, a facility to conduct the program in, etc.

The health committee may also decide that because of limited resources, efforts may be better spent working with other community health groups. This may include helping to change various city health policies or laws, or working with local media groups to get certain health messages across to the entire community. Or committee members may choose to provide certain health services at local schools, health departments, hospitals, or worksites that have the finances and facilities to support such efforts.

Step 4—Before actually conducting a health program, it is recommended that some sort of health screening be done to determine the level of health in participants. Screening programs serve two purposes: to assess the prevalence of risk factors and attract large numbers of people.

Four types of screening programs are recommended as the most practical: (1) measurement of serum cholesterol with portable analyzers; (2) measurement of blood pressure; (3) computerized assessment of several health practices including diet, overall health risk (health risk appraisal), and stress levels; (4) measurement of body fat using appropriate equipment.

Management of the entire screening program requires the leadership of a health professional who adheres to standard screening practices. All participants in the screening program should fill out a medical/health questionnaire that allows the health leader to carefully determine the most pressing needs of the group.

Step 5—Based on the results of the screening programs, the medical/health questionnaire, and the viewpoints of community health leaders, the health committee can identify the major health needs of the group or community participants. These can be listed and prioritized according to importance, and the various health programs planned.

For example, high stress and high blood pressure levels may be determined as the most prevalent health problems in the group that was screened, followed by cigarette smoking and obesity. The committee can discuss community and environmental factors that may be influencing some of these problems, as well as barriers some participants may have in their desire for change. Based on all the information, the health committee can plan the health programs.

Step 6—The health committee next organizes and implements the health programs. These may include stress management seminars, weight control programs, cooking schools, smoking cessation programs, walking-fitness groups, or heart disease prevention classes. It is a good idea to link health screening with specific health programs that are designed to help high-risk individuals develop improved health habits.

Step 7—The final step, which is actually an integral part of the entire health promotion process, is evaluation. The health committee should carefully consider all the data collected during all phases of the process, learn from both successes and mistakes, and use the information to move ahead with better plans for the future.

How Can Participants Be Led to Christ?

This is a difficult question that each church group will have to answer, applying certain principles to their unique circumstances. Some of the issues discussed in chapters 1 and 10 may be especially valuable in deciding how to approach this challenge.

One of the core principles, as explained by Ellen White, is "wise restraint." "Let our consistent lives win confidence and awaken a desire to know why we believe as we do. . . . Do not allow them to receive an impression that you are intensely anxious for them to understand and to accept our faith. It is natural that there should be an intense fervency to this end. But often a wise restraint is necessary. . . . Not *words*, but *deeds*. . . . A uniform cheerfulness, tender kindness, Christian benevolence, patience and love will melt away prejudice" (*Evangelism*, pp. 539-540, 543).

In others words, serve the participants in community health programs in Christian love, and soon they will start asking questions. Christ is our best example in this regard. "During His ministry, Jesus devoted more time to healing the sick than to preaching. His miracles testified to the truth of His words, that He came not to destroy, but to save" (*The Ministry of Healing*, p. 19).

The Adventist Healthstyle

Vibrant Life

Improve and protect your health with *Vibrant Life* magazine. It contains well-researched articles on fitness and nutrition and the latest information on medical breakthroughs. Colorful and easy to read, it comes with a Christian perspective that recognizes the connection between physical, emotional, and mental health, and faith in God. Send for *Vibrant Life* today, and discover a source of health information you can trust. One year (6 issues), US$8.97, Cdn$16.88.

Going Meatless

This special issue of *Vibrant Life* brings you the latest research information on vegetarianism. Special features include a nutrition chart giving you the daily requirements for a sound vegetarian diet, vegetarian recipes, and a list of popular vegetarian restaurants around the country. US$2.50, Cdn$3.00.

Fabulous Food for Family and Friends

If you love to entertain but value a wholesome diet, this cookbook gives you 18 full-course menus that bring sumptuous heart-healthy spreads to your table with elegance and style. More than 130 recipes provide that extra-special touch to a wide variety of occasions. By Cheryl Thomas Caviness. Spiral bound, 128 pages. US$10.50, Cdn$13.15.

Quick and Easy Cooking

Cheryl Thomas Caviness has created 24 complete meals that you can make (including the drink) in 50 minutes or less. Recipes are low in cholesterol, saturated fats, salt, and sugar, and eliminate meat and meat substitutes. Spiral bound, 112 pages. US$10.50, Cdn$13.15.

To order, call **1-800-765-6955** or write to ABC Mailing Service, P.O. Box 1119, Hagerstown, MD 21741. Send check or money order. Enclose applicable sales tax and 15 percent (minimum US$2.50) for postage and handling. Prices and availability subject to change without notice. Add 7 percent GST in Canada.